digestion

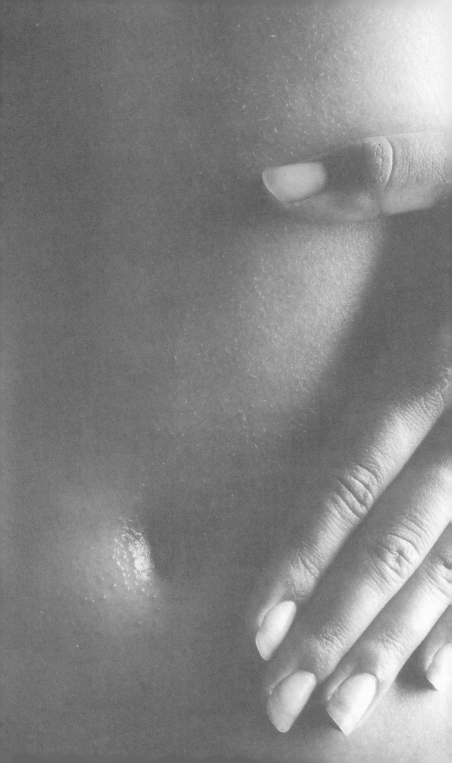

digestion

your 100 questions answered

Dr. Joan Gomez

Newleaf

First published by

NEWLEAF

an imprint of

GILL & MACMILLAN LTD

Hume Avenue, Park West, Dublin 12

with associated companies throughout the world

www.gillmacmillan.ie

ISBN 0 7171 3267 6

A CIP catalogue record for this book is available from the British Library.

Note from the publisher
Information given in this book is not intended to be
taken as a replacement for medical advice. Any person with
a condition requiring medical attention should consult a
qualified medical practitioner or therapist.

This book was conceived, designed and produced by
THE IVY PRESS LIMITED

ART DIRECTOR Peter Bridgewater
PUBLISHER Sophie Collins
EDITORIAL DIRECTOR Steve Luck
DESIGNER Jane Lanaway
PROJECT EDITOR Georga Godwin
DTP DESIGNER Chris Lanaway
MEDICAL ILLUSTRATOR Michael Courtney

Printed in Spain by Graficomo, S.A.

Contents

Introduction

As the means of turning food into the nutrients and energy you need you rely on the efficient functioning of your digestive system for your very existence. It consists of a string of very different parts that work as a team – each organ depending on the others – and the wonderful thing is that they need no servicing and never wear out.

The digestive system is unique in this durability. Our bones become thinner and may develop osteoporosis over time and muscles lose their strength, cutting short the careers of footballers and athletes. Your hair cannot go on indefinitely making its pigment, and if you are a man you may lose it altogether. Your skin becomes paper thin and fragile – but although your digestive system has to work day in and day out, never knowing what you will throw at it, it performs the miracle of turning the food on your plate into brain, brawn and bones when you are 80 just as well as it did 60 years before. The Queen Mother's century-old equipment can still deal with a State banquet!

A remarkable feature of the digestive system lies in its controlling and co-ordinating mechanisms. One of these is a network of nerves operating automatically and linking each area with the rest; the other comprises hormones and other chemical messengers that are carried round in the bloodstream so that each part or organ can pick up what it, individually, needs. This is the Internet system for the world of your body.

Although it does not suffer from plain wear and tear, such a complex set of arrangements must sometimes go wrong. It is fine to know what marvellous digestive apparatus you have – but your main concern, naturally, is that it should work smoothly. An essential aid is the warning system – the symptoms. They are the equivalent of a red light showing on the dashboard of your car, and they, too, remind you to take action: first to find out more, then, if necessary, to go to the doctor's.

Pain: this is the red alert, the most insistent of the warning signals, and one that will not let you ignore it. Analyse it to get the maximum information to pass to your doctor. Where is it and does it radiate to other parts? How often do you get it, and how long does it usually last? What makes it better – or worse? Is it long-term or acute – and how severe?

One of the most common disorders is loss of appetite, which is more often than not to do with your state of mind rather than your body – both depression and anxiety, or even pleasant excitement can put you off your food. Local problems in your stomach and indeed most general debilitating diseases can also kill your appetite.

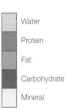

Water
Protein
Fat
Carbohydrate
Mineral

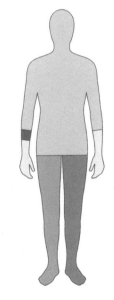

You are what you eat: your body is made up of types of the food that you eat. Here you can see the proportions of each.

Waterbrash: if your mouth suddenly fills with water, it tells you that something (not necessarily serious) is irritating the upper part of your gastrointestinal tract – gullet, stomach and duodenum. It could be a peptic ulcer, mild inflammation or the effect of an alcoholic drink.

Nausea: this means feeling sick and is usually, but not always, the precursor to vomiting. You want to lie down and keep your head low. One of the most distressing and persistent types of nausea, often lasting for several days, is a reaction to anti-cancer medication (that containing platinum is the worst).

Vomiting: this is normally preceded by nausea. It occurs in any acute problem in the digestive system, for instance, infection with bacteria or the presence of their toxins; chemical poisons or poisonous fungi; bad food – or blockage of the intestine or the outlet from the stomach, the pylorus. Very young babies may have pyloric stenosis, which makes them vomit constantly (until treated surgically). An infection anywhere is likely to cause vomiting in a child. For adults, too, there are conditions outside the digestive system that can cause vomiting, ranging from meningitis to migraine, and even some common drugs. Early morning vomiting should make you think of pregnancy, alcoholic excess or anxiety – particularly when it occurs on an important day in your life. Late evening vomiting, especially of a large quantity, suggests a blockage at the pylorus. Vomiting that is welcomed, because it relieves stomach pain, is usually due to a duodenal ulcer, but occasionally to a peptic ulcer elsewhere. Sudden vomiting without nausea may be due to direct irritation of the vomiting centre in the brain, for example in meningitis, stroke or a tumour, which may be benign or occur after a head injury. Vomiting causes a rapid loss in weight – a reason why girls with bulimia make a habit of it. If there is persistent vomiting with no loss of weight you can be sure there is a psychological cause. It is important to sort this out because the body chemistry can be disrupted.

Heartburn: this tells you that your oesophagus is inflamed – from burning hot food, undiluted spirits, excess of spices, or, commonly, from reflux of fluid from the stomach, including its acid. Sometimes the muscle contractions in the wall of the gullet get out of phase and give you a sensation like heartburn: typical of irritable bowel syndrome.

Regurgitation: food you have swallowed comes back into your mouth without effort or any feeling of nausea, often with swallowed air. It may mean that you have eaten rather too much, or it can be a bad habit – either way it is not a sign of anything wrong.

Dysphagia: difficulty in swallowing. This must always be checked out. It can be due to an enlarged thyroid gland, an aneurysm of the aorta, enlarged lymph glands or a lung tumour pressing on the gullet from outside. Inside the oesophagus there may be swelling round a peptic ulcer, or scarring from an ulcer or inflammation producing a narrow section:

stenosis. Disorders of the nervous system such as motor neurone disease or Huntington's chorea may make swallowing difficult.

'Wind': this comes from gas produced by bacteria in the colon and from swallowed air coming through the system. It is uncomfortable but not significant, and is one of the many symptoms of irritable colon.

Constipation: only four people in 100 have a bowel movement less than three times a week in the UK. This is one measure of constipation. The usual criterion, however, is having motions that are hard and difficult to pass. Constipation is an important symptom in the over-50s because of its sometimes being the early warning of the commonest cancer in the digestive system – colorectal cancer. It is also the forerunner of diverticular disease, and always occurs in blockage of the intestine. Usually, it means nothing more than a need for more dietary fibre.

Diarrhoea: apart from short-lived gastroenteritis, this is uncommon, but is associated with ulcerative colitis and one type of irritable bowel syndrome.

Loss of weight: this may be due to a reduced intake of nourishment, impaired appetite or anorexia nervosa; vomiting; or malabsorption and loss of protein in Crohn's disease and ulcerative colitis – but cancer anywhere in the body also leads to weight loss.

The appearance of symptoms may seem alarming, but they are a safety mechanism, telling you when there is a threat to your health, so that you can take avoiding action or zap a disorder that has started up.

Prevention

Although most people are likely to suffer from digestive upsets from time to time, there are steps that can be taken to prevent problems occurring – or at least to limit their severity and frequency. This section looks at how the digestive system actually works and at the dietary measures that will encourage it to function at its best. Prevention rather than cure is the aim.

The creation of energy is the result of the orderly activity of a series of co-ordinated organs – your digestive system.

It starts in your mind when you begin to think about food, triggered by the smell or the sight of it, or the clock indicating lunchtime. The saliva glands in your mouth are immediately producing their lubricating liquid and the enzyme, ptyalin, which is used in the digestion of carbohydrates. Next in line is your oesophagus or gullet which conveys the food and drink from your mouth to the collecting bag, the stomach. This is not a simple matter of gravity. The muscles in the wall of the oesophagus massage the contents on their way, so that a circus performer can drink a glass of water standing on his head.

The stomach muscles thoroughly mix everything that has arrived there before pushing it on into the duodenum. In the stomach hydrochloric acid and pepsin soften, sterilize and digest protein and carbohydrate – such foods as meat and two vegetables. In the duodenum, bile from the liver and pancreatic juice are added to the mix, and deal with the fatty foods. The task of the small intestine – all 22 feet of it – is to complete digestion and absorb the useful nutrients from the resulting chyme. This is vital work, without which the rest of the digestive system would be a waste of space.

The colon, or large bowel, receives the undigested liquid remains from the small intestine, and reabsorbs some of the fluid so that the motion becomes progressively thicker, from mushy to porridgey to firm and formed. The colon stores this material until enough has accumulated in the rectum, the last part of the large bowel, to stimulate it. You then get an urge to go to the lavatory, and the process is completed.

2 What is the difference between gastritis and gastroenteritis?

Gastritis, broadly, involves only the stomach, the collecting bag for food where a major part of digestion takes place. Gastroenteritis includes the whole of the digestive tract, both stomach and the intestines, small and large.

Gastritis is a term often used by lay people to refer to dyspepsia, but gastritis is a specific disorder, or group of disorders, characterized by inflammation of the stomach. It may be acute – short-lived and severe – or chronic, a long-term problem. Acute gastritis may be due to swallowing an irritant, for instance aspirin, but is more often caused by alcohol (too strong and too much). The effects are at their worst the morning after a drinking bout: nausea, stomach pain and vomiting. Some illnesses with a high fever, such as influenza, can bring on gastritis.

Chronic gastritis is very common in the elderly. It may not cause symptoms, or there may be indigestion preventing the enjoyment of meals. Animals do not get this and no one knows why we do. It is occasionally the forerunner of stomach cancer. Infection with the bacterium helicobacter pylori is a common cause of chronic gastritis with pain and dyspepsia, and there is also an autoimmune variety of gastritis, one of the disorders in which the body's defences attack certain of its own cells.

Gastroenteritis is food-poisoning. It involves inflammation of both stomach and intestines. The symptoms are abdominal pain, vomiting and diarrhoea, as the body tries to rid itself of the noxious material. The infective causes include salmonella and Escherichia (E.) coli, and the non-infective includes chemical and fungal poisons.

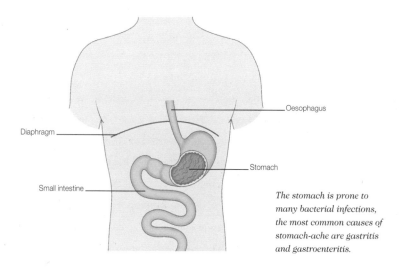

The stomach is prone to many bacterial infections, the most common causes of stomach-ache are gastritis and gastroenteritis.

Oesophagus

Diaphragm

Stomach

Small intestine

This depends on the cause. Food-poisoning falls into two types: those due to an infection and those with a non-infective cause. In general, hygiene around food preparation and the actual meals is helpful. This includes protective clothing, hand-washing and the use of tongs for workers in the food industry, ridding shops and kitchens of flies, and the habit of hand-washing after going to the toilet and before meals, inculcated in our children by adult example. Cooked and raw meats should be stored separately, all food should be refrigerated when possible, thoroughly defrosted before cooking and covered when it is in the open. Cooking, especially of meat, should be long enough to kill any organisms, making a rare steak off-limits. Seniors, young children and pregnant women need to take meticulous care in their food hygiene.

A number of different germs can cause food-poisoning: salmonella infection is very common. The risks come from inadequately defrosted or under-cooked chicken, and under-cooked or raw egg (as in mayonnaise). Carriers who handle food may pass the infection on, but thorough cooking counteracts this. Campylobacter is on the increase, affecting those who work with poultry or have a dog, and also from drinking contaminated water or unpasteurized milk. Children are especially susceptible. Listeria lives in soft cheeses and poultry. Babies, pregnant mothers, diabetics and alcoholics are at most risk. Some germs produce a toxin which causes food-poisoning. These include staphylococci, which are widespread germs, found on the skin, and passed on through handling food or food left uncovered. Clostridium botulinus, the cause of botulism, is rare and deadly and develops in damaged tins or preserved fish. Check your tins, and discard any that are doubtful.

Non-infectious causes include allergy, for instance to shellfish or strawberries. Certain Asian and tropical fish, especially raw, may be toxic. The food will seem perfectly fresh so it is impossible to know if it is safe; you have to take a chance. Some fungi, such as the Death Cap, are highly poisonous and are a danger if you pick your own 'mushrooms'.

4 What raw materials – food and drink – can the digestive system handle?

Keeping your body going – muscle work, talking, thinking, and so on – requires a constant source of energy. The fuel to supply this is food, which you burn like any other fuel, but slowly – although you feel warmer after a meal. Just as a car cannot run on coal, so you require a special type of fuel. It consists of three classes of nutriment: carbohydrates, fats and proteins – we can use those from either animal or plant sources, being omnivorous (rather than carnivorous or herbivorous, like a lion or a rabbit).

Although your digestion can cope with an enormous variety of foods, it cannot digest plant fibre. The appendix is a useless vestige of the organ that deals with it in horses. You also need a mixture of foods from the different classes for digestion to work – hence such dishes as fish and chips or meat and two vegetables. Gimmicky slimming regimes that restrict you to one type of food cause a temporary loss of weight by disabling your digestion.

Drinks that contain caffeine – coffee, tea and cola – like cigarettes, impair digestion: one reason why reformed smokers put on weight and obsessive tea or coffee drinkers are often thin. Alcohol in small quantities can aid digestion, but larger amounts and undiluted spirits inflame the digestive system.

Some foods are poisonous, although they may look all right. Your senses of smell and taste will warn you if meat or milk is 'off', so that you can spit it out. When the poisonous nature of food is not obvious, for example rhododendron honey, the stomach may reject it and you vomit, and with some bacterial poisons you can get diarrhoea.

Salmonella and Clostridium are two of the more well-known bacteria which live in food and if consumed can cause 'food poisoning'.

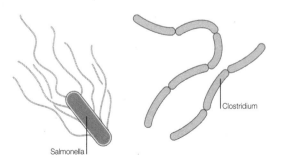

Salmonella

Clostridium

Q

5 I keep reading about a 'balanced' diet. What does this mean?

A balanced diet is one comprising the correct proportions of protein, fat and carbohydrate foods to provide for your needs: growth in pregnancy and childhood, and the repair and continuous replacement of your tissues at any stage, and the energy for all your activities. It should also supply the tiny amounts needed of vitamins and minerals. The only supplements likely to be required are of iron or calcium, in the over-40s, folate in pregnancy and vitamin B_{12} in vegans.

Nutritionists in Western countries have all set out similar national guidelines for a balanced diet. The UK diet recommends that one-third of the intake should consist of fruit and vegetables, one-third of bread, rice, cereals and potatoes, with the rest divided between meat, fish and alternatives, and low-fat dairy products, plus a small quantity of sugary and fatty foods. The official Canadian advice is to take, every day, something from each of four groups: milk and milk products, meat and alternates, bread and cereals, fruit and vegetables. Guidelines from the United States National Research Council, and from the other authorities, are as follows: reduce your total fat intake to 30 per cent of

This piechart shows the proportions of the types of food you need to have a balanced diet. You should eat a variety of foods from each group every day.

Fruit and vegetables

Bread, cereal, potatoes

Meat, fish and alternatives

Fats, sugary foods

Milk, dairy foods

your total calories; fat from animal sources should be no more than 10 per cent; eat fish regularly; eat five or more helpings of fruit and vegetables daily, especially the green and orange kinds; eat six or more servings of bread, cereal, and legumes daily; take only a moderate amount of protein: about 56g daily for men, 45g for women; do not add salt to your food and drink alcohol only in moderation (two drinks daily for men, and just one for women).

6

What is the difference between a vegetarian and a vegan diet? Can either of them be harmful?

Vegetarianism is increasingly fashionable, partly on kindness-to-animals grounds, partly because some people believe it is healthier and more natural. Whether it is healthy or not depends on the level of vegetarianism. We can distinguish the following stages or degrees. First, cutting out some meats for cultural reasons, for example horsemeat. This applies to most British and Americans and constitutes a normal diet. Second, no meat or poultry, but fish and dairy products allowed. With this there is little risk of running short of any particular nutrient. Third, no meat, poultry or fish, but milk products and eggs allowed: a lacto-ovo-vegetarian diet. This is standard vegetarianism and the main risk is a lack of iron. Fourth, a vegan diet; no animal products of any kind allowed. Vitamin B_{12} deficiency is likely, affecting every cell in your body, causing a serious form of anaemia, intractable back pain and mental disturbances in the over-40s, and is extremely dangerous in children. You may also lack calcium, iron and zinc. Blue-eyed women are particularly susceptible. Fifth, a fruitarian diet: an attempt to live on fruit alone always fails. You run short of protein, vitamin B_{12}, all the fat-soluble vitamins and most of the minerals you need.

A moderate vegetarian diet can reduce the risk of coronary heart disease, high blood pressure, obesity, and possibly some cancers. It is not recommended for pregnant or breast-feeding women and growing children, who all do better with some animal protein. Protein is the main problem if you are a vegetarian, and you have to plan your meals carefully to include plenty of legumes (including soya) and nuts to supply essential amino-acids.

In 1833 William Beaumont discovered, in a patient with a gunshot wound opening into his stomach, that the movements and the amount of acid produced varied with the man's emotional state. This is the first of several considerations when you want to make the conditions favourable for the digestion of your meal. If you are upset or stressed, then it is better to postpone a main meal and settle for a milky drink and a plain biscuit. This combination quietens the stomach, putting no strain on it. A period of unwinding before supper also makes good sense.

Regularity tunes in with your bodily rhythms. Your stomach, like your heart, has a pacemaker. It runs in cycles of 90–120 minutes. That is why we get an urge to have coffee halfway between meals. If you can keep to your usual meal times on holiday, stomach upsets are less likely. Block off at least half an hour for a meal to allow digestion to get under way. It can upset your digestion if you take vigorous exercise, like swimming, within an hour of a main meal. Company at meals is beneficial because it is relaxing, wiping out work problems and preventing your eating too quickly. Radio, TV or a book can serve the same purpose.

Where you eat matters, too. If you eat sandwiches at your desk or a burger on site, your body will not get the message that digestion is top priority now and the circulation to your stomach needs boosting.

Consider your posture. Sitting upright in a dining chair is ideal for your stomach. Lounging on a low sofa watching TV or balanced on a bar-stool can crease your stomach, while constricting belts impede its churning activity.

I learned at school that digestion begins in the mouth. What does this mean and how can I help this process?

As soon as there is food in your mouth the taste buds on your tongue assess it from a mix of four basic tastes: sweet, sour, salty and bitter. The taste buds at the front of your tongue are especially sensitive to sweetness; those at the back to bitterness. An acceptable flavour sets off a reflex in the salivary glands and they pour out their fluid. Meanwhile you begin chewing: your front, incisor teeth bite off a chunk of food and the grinders smash it up. Then it is mixed with saliva to form a bolus, a soft lump of food the right size to swallow. The salivary glands lie under your tongue and jaw, and over the angle of the jaw. They produce two kinds of saliva, watery or serous, and mucus. The serous type contains ptyalin, an enzyme that converts starchy foods into maltose, a sugar. You cannot take a doughnut directly into your bloodstream, but a sugar solution is absorbed immediately. If you chew a piece of bread for several minutes you taste the sweetness. Normally, you only keep food in your mouth for about one minute, but the ptyalin goes on working in the stomach. Ptyalism is a term given to an excessive production of saliva, and occurs when the stomach is irritated. You can help your mouth at work by following Gladstone's advice to chew your food 32 times, by finishing your meals with fruit, cleaning your teeth especially at night, and having six-monthly dental check-ups.

I keep hearing that we should eat more fibre. Why do we need it and what sort of foods contain fibre?

Fibre is the indigestible part of your food, making up the bulk of your motions. Yet it is important to the health of your digestive system, specifically your colon. This can only work with enough food residue inside it to stimulate the muscle. Modern diets of refined, processed products provide neither bulk nor the mechanical stimulus of slightly coarse material passing through. Lack of fibre leads to constipation and thereby increases the likelihood of diverticulitis or colon cancer. A high-fibre diet, recommended by nutritionists throughout the West, reduces the risk of these disorders, obesity and, in some cases, irritable bowel syndrome. If you eat plenty of soluble fibre, your cholesterol level will be reduced, a protection against coronary heart disease. Fibre is an integral part of plant structure and includes pectins (which make jam set), lignins and cellulose. There are two types, soluble and insoluble. Soluble fibre occurs in oats, oat bran and legumes, while wheat bran and wholemeal provide insoluble fibre The official recommendation is to eat 20–30 grams of fibre daily: a minimum of five portions of fruit and vegetables and six of wholemeal bread and cereals. Good sources include cornflakes, puffed wheat and bran cereals; prunes and dried apricots; frozen peas; desiccated coconut. Fibre supplements are available, but fibre from food has fewer side-effects.

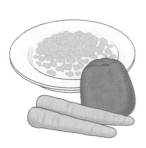

High-fibre foods such as fruit, root vegetables and cereals can help maintain a healthy digestive tract.

In spite of government and medical pressure to eat more fibre, not everyone can tolerate a high-fibre diet, especially if over the years they have been accustomed to low-residue foods such as crisps, white bread, cakes and biscuits. If you plan to increase your fibre intake considerably, take your time. Gradually introduce sieved or puréed, cooked vegetables and fruit. Little by little add unsieved food, then raw fruit and vegetables, grated at first.

The side-effects of fibre, which can be intolerable, include flatulence, bloating and cramps, surprisingly diarrhoea is a less common effect. These symptoms are sometimes part of irritable bowel syndrome or diverticulitis, in which case you must find out which fibre-rich foods and in what quantities your bowel will tolerate. Bran, particularly wheat bran, is probably most likely to cause troublesome side-effects, but much worse are laxatives based on fibre. The severity of the side-effects depends on your constitution. If you suffer from megacolon (an oversize colon), it is harmful to fill it with fibre. If you have hard motions that have got stuck, it is dangerous to add fibre to the problem – even more so if you have a threatened blockage, as in ulcerative colitis, Crohn's disease or diverticulitis. If you increase your fibre intake, it is essential also to *increase your intake of water*.

It is a pleasure to have a good appetite and to see your child eating well. How can you stimulate an appetite, for instance after an illness?

A good appetite means looking forward to your meals, expecting to enjoy them, based on your previous experience. Young children are 'picky' because so many foods are strange to them. As an adult your environment and the company count for more than your physiological need for nourishment. The smell and taste of food often stimulate appetite. A simple cold in the head makes your food seem unattractive because your sense of smell is impaired. You 'spoil' your appetite by having a snack shortly before a meal, but it is put out more seriously in illness, especially if this involves pain or a fever. Too much alcohol, once-off or long-term, douses your appetite, and a whole range of medicines do the same, including some herbal remedies. If you are depressed or anxious you may not want to eat.

It is worrying when someone who has been ill, especially your child, loses their appetite, but fresh air and gentle exercise are helpful. Avoid stodgy or dry foods without much flavour, and greasy and highly spiced dishes. Light, easily digested meals in small helpings go down best: for example, scrambled egg instead of steak and kidney, fruit yoghurt rather than Black Forest gateau. Six small meals a day stimulate the appetite twice as much as three substantial meals, while missing a meal does not increase your appetite for the next one.

Q

12 I feel hungry when I sit down to a meal but after a few mouthfuls I feel full up. What is the cause of this?

It is common to feel uncomfortably full after a meal – at its simplest, you may have eaten too much and some foods make you feel full sooner than others. What is disconcerting is discomfort when you have hardly eaten anything. This occurs in anorexia: the stomach has adjusted to tiny meals by shrinking. Much the same occurs with gastric stapling to make the stomach smaller as a slimming ploy. Hiatus hernia, in which your food goes back into the oesophagus instead of the stomach, also produces undue fullness. The usual cause, however, is faulty nervous control of the muscles of the stomach and colon. Normally, as soon as food enters the stomach, its regular, between-meals rhythmic activity switches off and is replaced by the digestive routine. Special mixing contractions begin, combined with gentle propulsion towards the duodenum, the adjoining part of the alimentary tract. If this pattern does not kick in, the food does not move on and stomach muscles tighten up, or contract irregularly. Often the large bowel is also involved. When food arrives in the stomach a message is flashed to the colon, setting off a muscular movement towards the anus. If this does not happen you may get a reaction of bloating. Over-fullness after food can be a symptom on its own or part of the irritable colon syndrome, diverticular disease or dyspepsia of the non-ulcer kind.

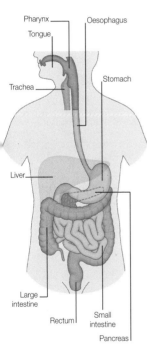

Pharynx

Oesophagus

Tongue

Trachea

Stomach

Liver

Large intestine

Rectum

Small intestine

Pancreas

Food passes down your oesophagus into your stomach. From there it makes its way past your pancreas and small intestine, large intestine and rectum before the waste is expelled through your anus.

Alcohol is poison in large quantities – acute alcoholism can kill you – and an irritant in smaller amounts. It affects every part of the digestive system. The pleasant, warm glow as you swallow a mouthful of spirits is, in fact, a wave of inflammation passing down your oesophagus into your stomach. Acute gastritis often follows a drinking bout, and steady drinking causes chronic gastritis. It greatly increases the risk of a duodenal ulcer or pancreatitis, acute or chronic. However, the prime target is your liver. Alcohol can cause fatty liver, alcoholic hepatitis and cirrhosis, a frequent cause of death. Irritation of the colon brings diarrhoea and, more seriously, the development of polyps and of cancer of the rectum.

There is no substitute for abstinence, but there are several ways of lessening the harmful effects. Avoid spirits, but if you must have them dilute them well with a non-fizzy liquid. Beer is especially likely to cause a fatty liver. Apple-based drinks – cider and calvados – are associated with rectal cancer. Fortified wines like sherry and port are almost as harmful as spirits, but ordinary red or white wine is the least damaging. Drinking only with your meals cuts down the risk, and a glass of milk forms a protective lining to your stomach. Avoid iron tablets. Wheat grain, bran, folate, the other B vitamins and vitamin C all tend to counter the effects of alcohol.

Q

14 How much should
a normal man or
woman eat,
measured in
calories?

Calories are a measure of the heat produced by a substance when it is burned: this equates with energy. Calories are a convenient way of comparing the energy values of different foods. Kilocalories (kcal, or just calories for short) are larger units to fit human usage. Whilst the average daily intake for an average man is around 3000 kcal, for women it is 2300 kcal (females actually require only 75 per cent of the calorie intake of males). The recommended average daily calorie allowances are:

CALORIE REQUIREMENTS (kcal)

Age group	Male	Female
Adult group, aged 19 to 59	2265	1751
Middle-aged group, aged 60 to 74	2355	1900
Seniors, aged 75 plus	2100	1810
The younger set, aged 15 to 18	2755	2110
Middle childhood, aged 7 to 10	1970	1740

Athletes need a much higher calorie intake than the average man or woman – they are capable of burning up to 8000 calories a day if, for instance, they are competing in strenuous activity such as the famous cycling race, the Tour de France! The calories that are used in different activities (kcal per hour) are shown below.

CALORIE REQUIREMENTS
DURING ACTIVITY

Activity	kcal per hour
Sleeping	70
Sitting	100
Standing	105
Keyboard work	115
Slow walk	200
Carpentry	240
Walking, golf, gardening	300
Tennis, cycling, swimming	420
Squash, jogging, hill climbing	600
Fast walk	700
Climbing stairs	900

Q

15 Which advice is right: to take three good meals a day with nothing in between, or to have small, frequent meals?

One thing is certain: grazing – that is, nibbling throughout the day – gives your digestion no peace and is always bad for you. A healthy adult does best with three meals, but a drink between them does no harm. It is also helpful to your digestive system to start the day with a hot drink.

Each of the three meals has a special importance. Breakfast, after the night-long fast, must include some speedily available energy, for instance from a breakfast cereal or from toast and marmalade, and some complex carbohydrate, such as some fruit, or a protein food, such as an egg, which releases its energy slowly.

Lunch should always include a significant protein component, but should not be heavy or indigestible as you need to be active during the afternoon. A tuna, ham or cheese salad with pasta, potato, or a roll or crispbread is suitable.

As for supper, since you are unlikely to undertake much muscle work to draw the circulation away from the digestive process during the evening, you can afford to indulge in richer foods at this meal, whether it be steak and kidney pie or a nut roast. You have all night to digest this meal. A word of warning, though – if you tend towards plumpness, every scrap that you eat at this meal will be digested and absorbed by your body.

Little and often are your watch-words if you have lost weight and need to build yourself up; if you are recovering from an acute illness; if you sometimes have digestive problems; or if you have a chronic illness or you are very senior – 90-plus. The meals must be bland, not fried or highly spiced, nor sweet and full of cream. They comprise breakfast, lunch and supper with snacks between and before bed.

16 Which foods and drinks should I avoid or minimize, to keep my digestive system healthy?

Avoid packaged food past its sell-by date or any food which, by smell, taste or age, you suspect of being 'off' – meat, shellfish (especially oysters), eggs and milk are likely offenders. Be wary of made up dishes that have been exposed to germs in the atmosphere. Trifles, custard, and egg concoctions are especially liable to harbour the staphylococci of food-poisoning. Damaged tins are a danger sign. Intrinsically poisonous foods like the Japanese puffer fish should be avoided; eating that is simply like playing Russian roulette. Fungi that have not been cultivated may also be deadly. Some Chinese foods, especially wonton soup, may cause the Chinese restaurant syndrome because of an excess of monosodium glutamate, causing burning in your trunk and shoulders as well as a headache. Be careful of any food that has caused a reaction in you previously: you may be hypersensitive or developing an allergy. Look out for inappropriate foods, for example Dundee cake for a toddler, or peanuts on which he may choke.

Cut down on junk food, which has little or no nutritive value in terms of protein and vitamins, but is often loaded with fat or sugar. Also reduce salt: restrict it to less than 6 grams daily. Do not add it to cooking or at the table, and beware of ham, sausage and soy or other sauces. Saturated fat from animal sources should be reduced. Currently it provides 15 per cent of our UK energy intake, but should be less than 10 per cent. Alcohol is an irritant to the whole digestive tract, with spirits and sherry the worst. Cola-type drinks can damage your teeth by dissolving the enamel. Bitter lemon can also cause problems, including haemorrhages into the skin.

17 I've heard that being overweight is worse for you than being underweight, yet fat people do not necessarily eat more. What is the explanation for these two facts?

In Western culture thin people have the edge, healthwise. They live longer and do not succumb as often to the diseases of our time – stroke, heart disease and, less seriously, arthritis. The problems due to overweight include cerebro-vascular disease (furring of the arteries to the brain), increasing the risk of death by 53 per cent; coronary heart disease, increasing it by 35 per cent; various cancers, increasing it by 16 per cent; diabetes, increasing the risk by 133 per cent; high blood pressure; chest diseases; gall stones; hernias; arthritis of the knees, hips and back; and varicose veins.

If you are overweight you are liable to develop sleep apnoea – a condition in which you repeatedly stop breathing in your sleep, waking you up all night. You are also likely to be more accident-prone and if you fall you damage yourself more because of the weight, with an increased risk of mortality of 18 per cent. Fat people may seem to eat very little (though of course they may stoke up in secret). This can be because the foods they choose look small on the plate but are highly calorific – butter on their bread, sugar in their tea, sausages instead of lean meat, chips or mash instead of salad, cake instead of fruit. They may choose chocolate or confectionery instead of an apple to finish a meal. Another factor is lack of exercise. A fat tennis player positions himself well but moves his body less than his opponent. Medical causes also exist. You may hope that the cause is an under-active thyroid, and sometimes it is. Steroid medication produces an appearance of fat, especially of the trunk and face, but the puffed-out tissue does not consist totally of fat.

You can eat more food providing you choose what you eat carefully – lots of fruit and vegetables, and take lots of exercise.

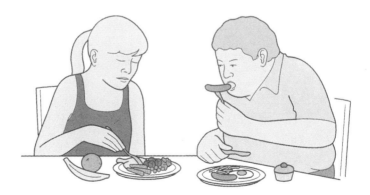

18 How should I modify
my diet during
pregnancy?

You do not actually need to eat more in
pregnancy. What you need are increases in
specific nutrients. Folate is the most urgent need to
insure against some nerve defects. A normal diet
may not supply the extra 220 micrograms you need
daily from conception. The best natural sources are
bran, endive, broccoli, spinach, avocado, egg yolk
and peanut butter. Liver contains plenty of folate but
sometimes dangerous amounts of vitamin A, so is
unsuitable. Iron is another must. Red meat two or
three times a week is far the most efficient source of
iron, but a vegetarian must take tablets. Calcium is
needed; half a litre (¾ pint) of milk or 60g (2oz) of
Cheddar cheese gives you 600mg (half of what you
need). Zinc is also necessary: you get it from meat,
wholegrain, shellfish, nuts and cheese. During the
growth of the foetus your thyroid uses more iodine,
but can take this from your normal diet. Protein is
essential building material for your baby's body, and
also for bigger breasts, the womb and the placenta.
You need an extra 10g, bringing the total daily intake
to 60g (2oz). Some must be from animal sources, but
you should avoid unpasteurized milk, soft cheeses,
pâté, raw egg and pre-cooked food.

Alcohol's effects start from conception. More than
one drink daily may cause foetal alcohol syndrome,
with physical and mental damage.

When things go wrong

Inevitably there are times when things go wrong with the body, and the digestive system is no exception. This section looks at ways of treating a first attack (and how to recognize it), at stomach and abdominal problems, ulcers and excretion and, finally, at tumours and cancer. There are measures that may be taken to alleviate all these conditions.

First attack

When digestive problems first occur they are often dismissed as a temporary problem or the result of overindulgence. But your body may be sending you subtle signs that something is wrong – perhaps you have an allergy or an intolerance to a particular food, perhaps your diet is not ideal for your way of life or that you are under too much stress and need to increase your intake of certain nutrients to counterbalance this. This section looks at the onset of digestive problems and how best to cope with them.

19 What is the difference between food allergy and food intolerance?

Food sensitivity involves having an adverse physical reaction whenever you eat a particular food or ingredient. The term allergy is often used loosely to mean almost any kind of food upset. True food allergy, however, occurs when an antigen or trigger in the food interacts with an immunoglobulin in the immune system. It can only happen if you have eaten the food before – unlike other sensitivities. Histamine is produced, setting off various types of symptom.

To test for a food allergy your doctor will perform a skin test showing the presence of the immunoglobulin. This, follwed by the laboratory analysis of a blood sample can pinpoint the exact food concerned.

Anaphylaxis is the most dangerous kind of allergic reaction, involving the breathing and circulation, and causing faintness and shock, with a dramatic fall in blood pressure. Symptoms of food sensitivity include swelling of the lips, diarrhoea and vomiting. There may be urticaria (nettle-rash) or eczema. You may have rhinorrhoea (a very runny nose) or asthma. Usually the reaction is acute and immediate, but it may be delayed, as in the case of coeliac disease, in which the victim cannot tolerate or absorb foods containing gluten (present in wheat).

Food intolerance includes reactions with no involvement of the immune system, mediated by other mechanisms – for instance, a lack of a particular digestive enzyme, lactase, causes an intolerance of milk. Some active chemicals may be present in the food: for example caffeine, causing a racing heart and tremor, or tyramine in some cheeses, causing a severe, throbbing headache. Pseudo-allergy means one of the allergic symptoms such as asthma, without an immunological input.

The timing of symptoms is variable. Swelling tissues, vomiting and rhinorrhoea appear within one hour. Nettle-rash and diarrhoea may take longer: 2–24 hours. Reactions lasting more than 24 hours include asthma and eczema. Some disorders may last for several days; these include headaches, irritability and general malaise. Long-term problems that may possibly be related to food include irritable bowel, hyperactivity disorder and migraine.

Q

20 Which foods can
cause allergies and
which can lead to
food intolerance?

Foods that commonly cause true allergic
reactions, including anaphylaxis (see Q 19), are
cow's milk; hen's eggs; peanuts (very dangerous);
fish, especially shellfish and oysters; wheat products;
legumes, especially peas and soya; fruits, especially
citrus, strawberries, apples and tomatoes; and
vegetables, for example, celery and peppers. You can
become allergic to almost any food, but food
intolerance has a wider range. Children are
particularly susceptible – up to 10 per cent of under-
10s are allergic to one of the foods on this list.

Different symptoms have different triggers.
Asthma in children is related to eggs, seafood and
nuts. In adults, it is related to flour, coffee, grains
and sulphur dioxide preservative. Infantile eczema is
related to eggs and milk. Flexural eczema (on the
elbows and knees) is related to milk, eggs and wheat.
In migraine there is usually a cumulative effect from
several triggers, plus food eaten some hours earlier.
Foods and drinks involved include chocolate, cheese
(especially cheddar and stilton) and red wine.

Acute urticaria (see Q 19) is related to foods that
release histamine, including strawberries, shellfish
and papaya. Foods containing histamine also include
some wines, fermented cheeses and sausages.
Chronic urticaria is linked to food additives such as
E numbers, benzoic acid and tartrazine in fruit

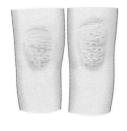

*Food allergies sometimes
show themselves as skin
disorders. Eczema of the
knees, for example, is a sign
of lactose intolerance.*

squashes, cordials, pickles, bottled sauces, salad cream, cake, soup and instant-pudding mixes, jelly, sweets, ice lollies, jam, curry powder, mustard and yoghurt. Vomiting and diarrhoea due to an immediate intolerance can occur when children taste a food for the first time – especially egg whites, nuts, milk or seafood.

Some uncommon sensitivities are to broad beans, causing anaemia; bitter lemon (containing quinine), causing skin rash; Chinese restaurant syndrome (from excess monosodium glutamate), causing headache, burning in the trunk and shoulders, and chest pain. A few people get headaches, palpitations or vomiting from tea or coffee.

21 What is an elimination diet and how does it actually work?

Elimination diets are a way of detecting the offenders in food intolerance or allergy. While you are on the diet you lose your symptoms. There are three phases. In the first phase the foods you normally eat are forbidden for three to four weeks. In the second, the foods are introduced one-by-one to identify which set off the symptoms. In the third (refurbishment), your diet is reorganized without the trouble-makers.

In the first phase you can have only water and sugar to drink. You can eat pears and lamb – or any combination of protein and fruit that you have not had often enough to develop a sensitivity to. You can choose a dozen foods instead of just two, but they must not include any that you eat regularly or alcohol, tea, coffee, herbal tea, sodas, chocolate, sweets, sugary foods, sweeteners, vinegar, pickles, highly spiced or salty food, sausages, pâté, curry, smoked fish or ham. You cannot have take-aways or café or restaurant meals. You must also avoid rare foods. This means the exotic foods that no one has often, such as paw-paw, truffles, caviare, tapioca, pomegranates, pine nuts, chickpeas, pumpkins and seeds, goose, rabbit or venison.

After the exclusion phase on one of these diets, comes the re-introduction, which takes seven to eight weeks. You try each of the excluded foods for two days running, watching for unpleasant symptoms – any you have had before, as well as headache, stomach-ache, feeling faint, nausea or vomiting. You can now identify the foods that are giving you trouble.

In the refurbishment phase you rebuild your diet along healthy lines, omitting the foods to which you are sensitive. You should include wholemeal bread, potatoes, brown rice, cereals without added sugar, milk, tuna, salmon, unsmoked fish, beans, lentils, green vegetables, salads, fruit and fresh meat.

Someone mentioned to me that aspirin might give me an upset stomach. Is this true and are there any other medicines which might have a similar effect?

Aspirin is a well-known stomach irritant. It causes erosions in the lining, which bleed and cause dyspepsia (the commonest and mildest effect). Acute, superficial ulceration occurs occasionally, and chronic peptic ulcer, gastric or duodenal, is an important reaction, but probably requires additional factors. Aspirin acts as a pain-killer by suppressing the production of prostaglandin, which causes pain and swelling of the tissues, and of mucus, which protects the stomach lining. Tablets and soluble aspirin are equally likely to cause symptoms, particularly if taken with alcohol. They can also cause nausea, vomiting and ringing in the ears (tinnitus).

Anti-inflammatory drugs, so helpful in arthritis, have a similar effect. Some heart drugs may cause adverse reactions in the digestive tract, while others for bowel inflammation and to reduce cholesterol can cause nausea and stomach pain. Iron tablets taken excessively can penetrate the thick layer of mucus covering the stomach membrane and cause dyspepsia. In extreme cases these may also cause constipation or diarrhoea, black motions or jaundice. Medicines that can cause diarrhoea, nausea and excess gas in the gut include some antibiotics, a few antacids, some medications taken for osteoporosis, and some laxatives, which may produce colic-like stomach cramps.

Q

23 I have been told
that I need tests to
'screen' my digestive
system. What does
this mean, and what
can I expect?

A screening test is carried out on people thought to be at risk of a particular disorder. If the problem is detected at an early stage, before it has caused definite symptoms, there is a good chance of curing it. Screening for breast cancer by means of a mammogram is a familiar example.

Rigid sigmoidoscopy – that is, passing a tube with a light in it into the back passage – is uncomfortable but not painful and is done with sedation. Barium enema, which shows up in X-ray and outlines the inside of the rectum and colon, reveals some problems that may be missed by the rigid sigmoidoscope. Even using both of these means of investigation, some colon disorders are not detected, so in some centres they use flexible sigmoidoscopy with fibre-optics, which gives a better view. An even better method, but requiring a very skilled operator, is colonoscopy, which allows detailed viewing of the whole of the colon and the facility for taking biopsies – that is, minute samples of tissue which can be examined microscopically. Gastroscopy is the only way of screening the stomach.

Blood tests are the commonest general-purpose screening tools. They involve no more than a needle prick. Examination of the motions detects several disorders and simply involves supplying a sample in a special container.

When I wake up
in the morning my
stomach is quite flat,
but as the day goes
on it gets bigger and
bigger, however little
I eat. Why does this
happen?

Lying in bed, your stomach is at its flattest, since it is able to relax to each side. Also, overnight you will have passed, imperceptibly, the gas in your bowel. The common, disconcerting experience is for the abdomen to start swelling immediately after your morning tea or breakfast – no matter what this consists of. The arrival of food in the stomach should set off the muscular movements in the system that facilitate digestion, but these may, instead, be irregular and uncomfortable. In an unconscious effort to relieve this, the abdominal muscles relax, allowing more bulging. What fills your abdomen is air or gas – nothing solid could have such a rapid effect.

Swallowed air is important. We all swallow some air, but some of us unconsciously gulp in more than others. While gas production in the gut and lack of muscle co-ordination are significant, another factor is excessive production of gas in the colon. The colon contains a large number of 'good' bacteria that ferment this residue, producing hydrogen, methane and carbon dioxide. The volume of gas you produce mainly depends on the types of food you eat. A high-fibre diet is not always beneficial, since it provides more material for the bugs to work on. Foods that produce excess gas are the cabbage family and legumes, as well as onions, leeks, garlic, fennel, turnips and poppy seeds.

Q

25 Does the way I feel
mentally affect my
digestion?

The two most important psychological
conditions are depression and anxiety, both of
which interfere with digestion.

Depression means a lowering of mood and slowing
up of all your mental and physical processes. It
shows itself in loss of appetite, in turn causing weight
loss. Food tastes like cardboard and it is hard work
swallowing it. You may force yourself to eat, but
there is no pleasure in it. Because of the sluggish
response of your stomach to the arrival of food, you
soon feel you cannot eat any more, and the food lies
in your stomach and feels heavy. Since digestion
does not get under way, you have twinges of
indigestion and may feel nauseous. If you have a
minor discomfort or pain – anywhere, but commonly
in the abdomen – it is intensified when you are
depressed. A touch of indigestion may translate into
a dull, persistent abdominal ache. It is then difficult
to know whether the pain is making you depressed,
or depression underlies your pain.

Anxiety is associated with tension in the gut
muscles, with spasms of pain that can double you up.
In an ongoing anxiety state your appetite may go
either way, from 'I couldn't face anything' to
compulsive wolfing down of food that you do not
enjoy. While constipation is characteristic of
depression, loose motions are likely in anxiety.

I've read that a person's personality can affect the symptoms of such illnesses as irritable bowel syndrome or diverticular disease. Is this true?

Some digestive disorders have a range of symptoms that vary over time and are influenced by your particular personality traits. Irritable bowel syndrome is considered to be a psychosomatic disorder, which means that it has a large psychological element. Possible symptoms include constipation, diarrhoea, abdominal pain, mucus in the motions, bloating, nausea and vomiting. There may also be headaches, poor sleep, back pain and constant tiredness.

Personality traits affect which symptoms predominate. Neuroticism is a tendency to experience even quite ordinary events and situations more intensely than other people: you find yourself often having to report symptoms to your doctor; or you may have various symptoms at the same time. With pessimism you cannot envisage getting better; with hypochondriasis you are constantly worried that your symptoms mean life-threatening disease. With introversion you are inward-looking and over-sensitive to normal physical sensations. Extraversion is just the opposite: the symptoms and your reactions are apt to be dramatic. Alexithymia is a trait in which you find it difficult to express emotions and can only talk about physical suffering. Bereavement frequently comes over as nagging pain, low in the abdomen.

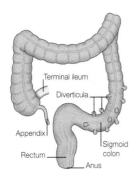

Terminal ileum
Diverticula
Appendix
Rectum
Sigmoid colon
Anus

Constipation caused by stress can lead to the development of small pouches in the colon called diverticular. Diverticular disease can be helped by a high-fibre diet.

I've noticed that my digestion is affected when I am under stress. How can I minimize this?

Stress is the bugbear of modern living, and your digestive system may be your Achilles heel. Stress results from too many demands on you; being boxed in by time constraints; financial stringency; threats to your home, health, job or key relationships; and physical stressors such as cold, fatigue, pain or infection. Breaks in routine are stress-savers – tea-breaks interrupt the vicious circle of stress and its symptoms. Coffee and tea in themselves are not ideal since they tend to increase anxiety and speed up the heart, but what is valuable is the 15-minute change of scene and thought.

Special care for your digestive system: do not eat at bedtime. The horizontal position does not suit the digestive process. And do not take vigorous exercise after a meal – it diverts blood from your stomach. During a working day, choose a light lunch, such as scrambled egg on toast; cheese, biscuits and fruit; or vegetable soup, a roll and an apple. Miss out all rich, spicy, fatty or super-sweet foods, red wine, strong coffee and cigarettes. Get enough sleep so that you wake easily and feel refreshed – and enough exercise. A minimum is three sessions of 40–60 minutes each week, preferably out-of-doors. Life events are a major source of stress, so avoid, if possible, two or more big changes (like marrying or moving house) within three months.

Why do I sometimes feel a 'lump' in my throat?

The feeling of a lump in the throat is a common experience, affecting up to 45 per cent of us at one time or another. Doctors often refer to it as 'globus', because it feels like a ball. You can get it at any age, but if you are under 50, it is three times as likely to occur if you are a woman. The characteristic feature is that, although the lump feels as big as a golf ball, it doesn't interfere with your swallowing. It often crops up when you are depressed or anxious, but in some cases it appears to come out of the blue, although a stressful situation may have been unconsciously suppressed and the globus symptom substituted. If you are conscientious, inclined to be introverted and obsessional about something, you are the personality type most liable to get globus. Understandably, you are likely to be concerned that something is wrong with your health. In fact, globus is uncomfortable but completely harmless, unless it prevents you swallowing.

For a few people great improvement follows the use of a tricyclic-type antidepressant, such as imipramine. This is most likely to help if you also have depressive or anxiety symptoms, affecting your mood, sleep and appetite. Relaxation exercises, including aromatherapy and yoga, may also help. Globus always recovers even without treatment, but it is likely to recur whenever you are under stress.

Difficulty in swallowing – dysphagia – is an important symptom and your doctor may send you to a specialist for further investigation.

There are several causes. There may be problems in the muscles or nerves of your pharynx, the part of your throat where the oesophagus and windpipe begin. The causes may be a hereditary nerve disorder, myasthenia gravis (progressive weakening of all the muscles) or inflammation of this area. The nerves rather than the muscles may be damaged – by polio, motor neurone disease, multiple sclerosis or Parkinson's disease. These disorders make it difficult to swallow either liquids or solids.

Stricture (narrowing) of the pharynx is uncommon and may be due to a harmless web of mucous membrane which is associated with chronic iron-deficiency anaemia. This develops very slowly and the symptoms come and go. More rapid development, with no let-up, can signify a cancer. Benign (harmless) or malignant (cancerous) strictures of the oesophagus are the commonest reasons for food sticking. Scarring may follow healing of an ulcer, making the stricture worse. Swallowing a corrosive poison also causes scarring. Cancer of the middle third of the oesophagus is the second commonest cause of dysphagia and is most likely to arise in your 60s.

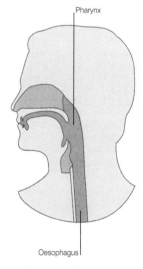

Pharynx

Oesophagus

After you have chewed your food the pharynx pushes it to the top of your oesophagus which in turn pushes it down into your stomach using a wave-like motion called peristalsis.

Recently I have been
vomiting a lot. I've
been told that it's
most likely a problem
with the upper part
of my digestive
system. Is this true?

Since vomiting is literally throwing up the contents of the stomach, it stands to reason that a common cause may be something wrong with the stomach itself or the oesophagus.

There are a number of possible causes. Peptic ulcers occur in the oesophagus, the stomach (gastric ulcer) or the duodenum (duodenal ulcer) close by. Nausea and vomiting may be the only symptoms, but usually you will also have pain and the vomiting provides a little relief. Cancer of the stomach often comes on with similar symptoms, but preceded in most cases by a severe loss of appetite. Gastritis – irritation and inflammation of the stomach – is commonly caused by alcohol, and sometimes by the nicotine of smoking, resulting in stomach-ache, nausea and vomiting. A number of medicines also has the side-effect of nausea and vomiting: for example some pain-killers, and chemotherapy drugs taken by mouth, as well as some medicines taken to combat digestive problems when taken incorrectly.

Oesophagitis due to inflammation from alcohol, spicy or physically hot food can

The main causes of stomach-ache are muscle spasm, ulceratins on the lining of the digestive system, gastritis and in some cases cancer.

Oesophagus

Area of spasm

Gastritis

Ulcer

Ulcer

Cancer

Duodenal ulcer

also cause vomiting. Hiatus hernia, bulging of the stomach into the oesophagus, may be responsible. Pyloric stenosis, narrowing of the entrance to the stomach, is a congenital abnormality in newborn babies, but in adults is usually the result of scarring from a peptic ulcer. It leads to evening vomiting. Post-gastrectomy syndrome may follow any stomach operation; you may get recurrent vomiting in the early morning and faintness after a meal. Gastroenteritis, due to food-poisoning, involves inflammation of the stomach and the intestines, and is due to staphylococci or other germs. Discomfort in the stomach and vomiting, usually followed by diarrhoea, come on four to six hours after a meal. The symptoms subside after 12–24 hours.

31 I often experience unpleasant nausea and vomiting, but there is nothing actually wrong with my stomach. What other problems can cause these symptoms, and how can I avoid them?

These symptoms may be due to disorders outside the digestive system. Severe pain, for instance, may indicate the agonizing colic of a kidney stone passing down the ureter, the tube to the bladder. To avoid the risk of kidney stones, drink plenty of water, particularly in hot weather or if you are sweating profusely. Stones in British people usually contain calcium or oxalate. Overload of calcium may be due to taking too much vitamin D, while oxalates come from fruit and vegetables, especially rhubarb, but it is only the latter that you need to consider.

A high temperature can lead to vomiting, especially in children. Drinking plain water increases the vomiting, so lemonade is better, with tepid sponging to keep the fever in check, since medicines like paracetamol may not be kept down. Infections affecting the bladder (for instance, cystitis) may cause vomiting in an elderly person as the first symptom. Throat and chest infections can have a similar effect, but you can only avoid them by keeping up your general health. Meningitis can cause severe vomiting, and where meningitis immunization is available, take it.

Pregnancy, especially in the mornings of the first three months, is a common cause. You can make vomiting less likely by taking plain biscuits with your early morning tea, and little between-meal snacks. Avoid getting tired.

Migraine may be set off by various foods, most often cheese, chocolate and red wine. Avoid whatever you know triggers it. There are also tablets you can take that act as a preventive. Head injury, especially if it leads to bleeding inside your skull, can cause sudden vomiting without any warning nausea, so have a check at a hospital after any head injury. An upset balance organ or a viral infection of the inner ear may also cause vertigo and nausea.

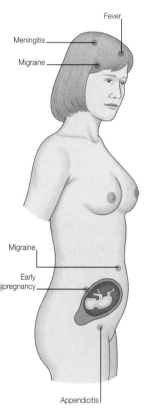

Fever

Meningitis

Migraine

Migraine

Early pregnancy

Appendicitis

Some of the main causes of vomiting excluding stomach problems include fever, meningitis, migraine, pregnancy and appendicitis.

32 Why is my tongue sometimes coated? I've been told this is due to constipation, but I am not constipated.

We all find our tongue coated from time to time, but it does not indicate any risk to health. Although it is said to be due to constipation, it has no connection with any abdominal disorder.

Smoking is the worst cause. If you are a regular smoker your tongue will frequently be coated, because smoking dries up the surface skin of the tongue, which becomes thicker and the little projections (papillae) stick up and harbour food particles, yeasts and bacteria. The long, filiform papillae at the back of your tongue are the most prominent and, since this part of the tongue is anchored, there is less chance of debris being washed away.

Mouth-breathing also dries the tongue. You get a hint of this if you accidentally go to sleep with your mouth open. Fever from any cause dries the mouth. Infection in the respiratory system does the same. Drinking milk and eating food that needs no chewing – for instance, custard or jelly – can cause coating.

Thrush (candidiasis) affects both babies and adults, the latter often after prolonged antibiotic treatment. Leukoplakia consists of white patches at first at the sides, then spreading over your tongue. It is not sore at first, but painful cracks develop. This condition needs urgent attention as it can be the forerunner of cancer.

I sometimes have
a sore tongue and
ulcers in my mouth.
Is this serious,
and what can I
do about it?

Neither a sore tongue nor mouth ulcers is serious in 99 per cent of cases. Glossitis (inflammation of the tongue), which looks smooth and red affecting the whole mouth. It is caused by a deficiency of iron or the group B vitamins: glossodynia is the name given to a persistently painful tongue, which looks normal and is not made worse by hot liquids. It is probably an emotional reaction, so you should check your lifestyle for stress. Aphthous ulceration is a common condition, but affects middle-aged women most often. The ulcers start as minute blisters and are very painful. Stress can precipitate an attack, and some women get them before their period.

Ulcers may be trivial, or severe and chronic if you have Crohn's disease, ulcerative colitis or coeliac disease. Hydrocortisone lozenges dull the pain, but you may need stronger steroid medicine by injection. Allergy or sensitivity to chemicals in toothpaste or dentures, and drugs, can also cause problems and require detective work to identify. Certain skin diseases, for instance lichen planus or pemphigus, may first appear in the mouth. Traumatic ulcers, due to badly fitting dentures, can be avoided by regular dental checks. If these ulcers persist for more than two weeks you need an investigation to look for other causes.

Q

34
I've been told that
the chest pain I
sometimes get is
connected with
my oesophagus. Is
this true? I thought
the oesophagus was
just a tube from my
mouth to my
stomach.

The oesophagus is not a simple tube. Its walls contain layers of muscle, whose task is to propel food from your mouth to your stomach by waves of contraction called peristalsis, taking eight to ten seconds to reach its destination. When you are upright, gravity speeds up the journey to five to six seconds. At each end of the oesophagus is a sphincter, a ring of muscle, which at the top closes off the food passage when you breathe, and at the lower end preventing reflux (flowing backwards of the stomach contents). The oesophagus is not sensitive, but when it hurts, in the chest, it is signalling damage. Peptic oesophagitis is inflammation of the oesophagus, usually due to failure of the lower sphincter to keep acid and digestive juices from harming the oesophagus lining. Peptic ulcer develops from this. Cancer may also occur, and there is a hereditary link.

Heartburn is a burning pain behind the breastbone. It is worse if you stoop or lie down and is caused by reflux.

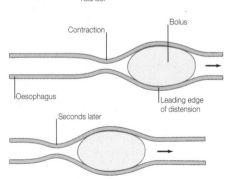

Oesophagus
Heartburn
Cancer
Ulcer
Cancer

Contraction
Bolus
Oesophagus
Leading edge
of distension
Seconds later

TOP *Common problems in the oesophagus include heartburn, ulceration of the inner membrane, and cancer.*
LEFT *Peristalsis works by pushing food along in a wave-like motion.*

Pain in the gullet (oesophagus) from heartburn is relieved immediately if you take an alkaline medicine, especially sodium bicarbonate. Peppermint tea also helps. Otherwise the best action (if you are inclined to plumpness) is losing weight. This reduces the pressure on the stomach that causes reflux oesophagitis (irritation of the lining of the oesophagus) if the stomach contents are squeezed upwards. Other types of peptic oesophagitis and ulcer also respond in the short-term to alkalis, but it is better to have a course of ranitidine or cimetidine from your doctor. Dyspepsia – indigestion, or pain associated with eating – may also be felt in the lower chest. Alkalis help, but in nervous dyspepsia a calm environment and, occasionally, a calming medicine are more useful.

To prevent pain in the gullet, do not smoke; moderate your alcohol intake and never drink spirits on an empty stomach; do not let your weight get more than 4 – 5lbs (2.5kg) over what is recommended for your height; avoid very hot, very cold and spicy food and drink. Do not eat large meals in the evening and avoid chocolate, fatty food, coffee, tobacco, alcohol and the medicine theophylline; they all relax the lower oesophageal sphincter, allowing reflux. Take a piece of soft bread and plenty of water when you swallow any tablets or capsules.

36 What causes a perforation – of the appendix, a diverticulum or any of the abdominal organs – and what are the effects?

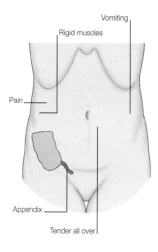

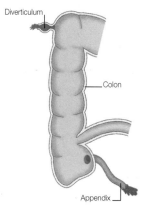

The causes of perforation, the breaking down of the wall of a viscus (a hollow organ) are twofold. First is a local weakening of the wall in one place, by infection running into suppuration: pus formation, as you see on a small scale in a boil. Second is an increase of pressure inside the organ. Underlying infection is important in peptic ulcer, diverticulitis and cholecystitis (gallbladder inflammation). Causes of increased internal pressure include obstruction of the gut by inflammation and scarring (for example, in Crohn's disease, gallstones), or impaction of something swallowed. It may also be caused by swelling of the contents of a viscus, for instance an ovarian cyst or an ectopic pregnancy. Severe injury to the abdomen (as in a traffic accident) can perforate an organ, and so can a medical accident during an endoscopic examination.

If perforation occurs, the contents of the organ erupt into the peritoneal space. This causes dramatic abdominal pain, so severe that any movement hurts. There is shock, with pallor, low blood pressure and shallow breathing. There is also tightening of the abdominal muscles to the point of rigidity.

TOP *The symptoms of appendicitis include pain on the right side of the abdomen.*
LEFT *The appendix and diverticulum are attached to the large intestine.*

Jaundice is a yellow discoloration of the skin and whites of the eyes (in French *jaune* = yellow). It is caused by a high level of bilirubin in the blood. Bilirubin is a breakdown product of haemoglobin from the red blood corpuscles. Worn-out blood cells are constantly being replaced, releasing bilirubin, which is converted into bile by the liver enzymes. It is stored in the gallbladder, then sent on to the intestine, finally being excreted in the motions, giving them their colour. When this mechanism goes wrong, bilirubin builds up in the bloodstream, causing jaundice.

Gilbert's disease is an entirely benign cause of mild jaundice, amounting to slight inefficiency in bilirubin disposal. Jaundice is not, in itself, harmful, but some of the reasons for it are serious. The basic causes are liver disease, blockage of a bile duct, and excessive breakdown of red blood cells. Viral hepatitis may be type A or type B. Type A, or infective hepatitis, is common among young adults. It has a long, vague incubation period, lasting six weeks to six months from contact with a case. It does not become chronic or lead to cirrhosis. Type B hepatitis is 'caught' through the mouth or by the bloodstream, for instance in a transfusion or between male homosexuals. It can become chronic. Glandular fever can also cause jaundice, as can some drugs.

Q
38 What are the
symptoms of
infective hepatitis?
Who is susceptible,
and what is the
treatment?

'Hepatitis' covers a number of illnesses in which there is inflammation of the liver and some liver cells die. The common causes are viral infections or various drugs, although poisonous fungi and solvents are occasionally responsible.

Hepatitis A, caused by the HAV virus, is often known as infective hepatitis. It is a self-limiting disease that runs a characteristic course with distinct phases. In the prodromal phase symptoms are loss of appetite, nausea and aversion to smoking in a smoker. There may be fever, headache and aching in the muscles, which may easily be mistaken for flu. An uneasy stomach and diarrhoea may be mistaken for gastroenteritis. A rash and joint pains may also occur. In the jaundice stage, the temperature settles, the urine is dark and the motions are pale.

The patient feels exhausted. In the recovery period the appetite returns and other symptoms subside. In post-hepatic syndrome there may be lethargy, depression and a feeling of being 'not up to par' for weeks.

Children are most often affected by hepatitis A, but adults most at risk are often young, healthy and intelligent. Bed rest is unnecessary, but you should avoid exhaustion. Fat in the food is traditionally forbidden, but this is unnecessary. No drugs actually help.

The liver can be prone to cirrhosis, hepatitis and some secondary cancer. Its function can also be affected by gallstones.

Cirrhosis

Secondary cancer

Liver

Gallstone

Hepatitis

Duodenum

Pancreas

The development of cirrhosis of the liver goes through four stages, each of which makes the abdomen get bigger. The first stage is fatty liver, when the metabolism of the liver is seriously disorganized, with droplets of fat in the liver cells. The liver is large, smooth and slightly tender. This is the 'beer belly' often seen on beaches, although it may be due to any kind of alcohol. The second stage is alcoholic hepatitis, a serious disease characterized by jaundice, a swollen liver, and the beginnings of an accumulation of free fluid in the abdomen. This is known as ascites. The third stage is cholestasis. It involves a failure of the liver cells to produce the normal flow of bile. Fluid builds up and the liver is more swollen and tender, enlarging the upper part of the abdomen, while there is more general abdominal enlargement as the ascites increases. Stage four is cirrhosis, when the liver becomes progressively harder and shrunken with the formation of scar tissue, leaving increasingly few healthy cells. The damaged liver retains sodium, adding to the fluid now distending the abdomen enormously.

There are a number of non-alcoholic causes of an enlarged abdomen, including obesity, pregnancy, bloating due to 'wind', osteoporosis and, more seriously, ovarian cysts, ovarian cancer, secondary cancers, primary liver cancer and even heart failure.

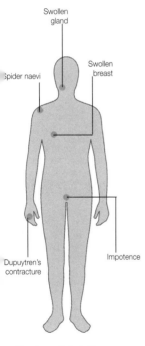

Swollen gland

Spider naevi

Swollen breast

Dupuytren's contracture

Impotence

The signs of alcoholism include swollen glands, swollen breasts in men, Dupuytren's contracture (see Q 40) and impotence.

Q

40 I have been told that I have Dupuytren's contracture and that it may be connected with my liver. What is Dupuytren's and what is the connection?

Dupuytren, an 18th-century French surgeon, first described this odd condition: a knobbly thickening and shrinking of the fibrous tissue that lies under the skin of your palm to strengthen it. This drags the fingers down, progressively, so that you cannot straighten them. Either or both hands may be affected, especially the fourth and fifth fingers.

Dupuytren's contracture may be associated with cirrhosis of the liver, usually (though not invariably) caused by long-term heavy drinking; however, it can also occur without any liver disease. The reason for the association with cirrhosis is not entirely clear, but cirrhosis involves the knobbly development of fibrous scar in the liver that can strangle the healthy liver cells. The liver is so important that when it is damaged the effects are felt all over the body.

Other symptoms that do not seem to be directly connected with the liver may occur in cirrhosis. Changes in the circulation cause spider naevi (groups of fine blood vessels in the skin); warm, red palms and a purply-blue nose. There may be hormonal effects, including loss of body hair and reduced interest in sex, and, in men, breast development, impotence and shrinking testicles. In women the breasts may shrink and menstrual periods reduce or cease; or a bleeding tendency may result in nosebleeds, heavy periods or spontaneous bruising.

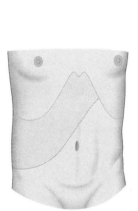

A disfunctional and enlarged liver can cause pain and discomfort in the abdomen, as shown here by the shaded area.

My doctor says I am
anaemic, but I eat
well and I have not
lost any blood. He
says I must have an
occult blood test.
What is this?

Your doctor may suspect that you are anaemic if you have several of the characteristic signs, including pallor, swollen ankles, lassitude, breathlessness when climbing stairs, palpitations, a throbbing sensation in your head and chest, ringing in your ears, headaches, poor sleep, pins and needles in your fingers and toes and chest pain. However, none of this proves anaemia, which can only be diagnosed by a blood test.

Iron-deficiency anaemia is the commonest type and is most likely to occur in disorders of the digestive system. In this, there is a reduced level of haemoglobin in your blood. The amount of iron in the plasma (the liquid part of the blood) is reduced, and the iron stores in the bone marrow are empty.

The most common reason for iron-deficiency anaemia is a chronic loss of blood through the digestive system – this may be either a slow, silent oozing or an intermittent bleed. It is detected by means of an occult blood test (occult means 'hidden'). You provide a sample of your motion, and then a tiny amount is put on a haemoccult slide. A blue coloration is a positive result, indicating blood loss from somewhere in the digestive system.

Common causes of such bleeding are a hiatus hernia, peptic ulcer, piles, cancer of the stomach or colon and certain drugs.

Dupuytren's contracture, a cramping of the inner tissue of the fingers causing them to curl under, may be caused by diseases of the liver.

Q

42 What is a PR? My doctor says he will do one next time I come to the surgery. What is it for and will it hurt?

PR stands for the Latin *per rectum* – via the back passage. It is the last part of a clinical examination of the abdomen. It is estimated that many lives would be saved if it were done as a routine. It is imperative if your symptoms point towards a problem in the colon or rectum, including changes in bowel habit, especially recent onset of constipation, bleeding from the back passage, prolapse (slipping out of part of the rectum), faecal incontinence and pain in the abdomen or anus.

Essentially a PR means the doctor feeling inside your back passage with a lubricated, gloved finger. You lie on the couch with a pillow under your hips and a blanket over you. The examination takes only a few minutes and, although uncomfortable, it is not painful – unless you have an anal fissure, an inflamed crack, in which case a local anaesthetic will help. PR allows the doctor to spot anal warts, abscess or haematoma, prolapsing piles, skin tags from Crohn's disease or leakage of motions, and to feel a chronic fissure or fistula polyps, abscess in the pelvis, 'foreign bodies', cancer of the rectum or gynaecological disease.

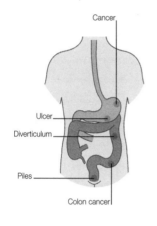

Cancer

Ulcer

Diverticulum

Piles

Colon cancer

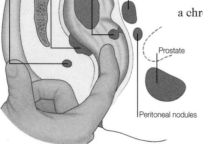

Rectal cancer

Lymph node

Polyps

Pelvic abscess

Prostate

Peritoneal nodules

A rectal examination (PR) can detect many diseases of the lower digestive tract including haemorrhoids, and tumours of the prostate gland and rectum (although it is impossible to tell whether these are malignant or benign).

43 I'm concerned
that my daughter
is suffering from
anorexia nervosa.
Is it true that it
is basically a
psychiatric
disorder?

Not every girl who is slimming suffers from anorexia nervosa. The criteria for the diagnosis are clear. Physically, loss of weight is the most striking feature. A weight of 4–5 stone (25–32kg) is not unusual, although parents are usually worried by anything less than 6st (38kg). The girl (it is a girl in nine out of ten cases) may disguise her appearance with baggy clothes, or flaunt her thinness. There is also often amenorrhoea (no monthly periods) for at least three months. There should be no known medical illness to account for the weight loss. The psychological criteria are a distorted body image (the girl sees herself as fat, even if she is skeletal), a refusal to keep to a normal weight, and an intense fear of putting on any weight.

The average age for anorexia to develop is 17–18 years, but it can begin as young as nine, and in a slightly different form at almost any adult age. Although the visible symptoms are physical, the driving force is emotional. The girl deliberately chooses a lifestyle calculated to reduce her weight, is obsessional about her diet, to the last calorie, and may develop an orange colour due to carotene from eating vast quantities of raw carrots. Obsessive exercising is another ploy for losing weight. She is constantly weighing herself, because she is terrified she will lose control and be unable to stop eating.

ANOREXIA NERVOSA

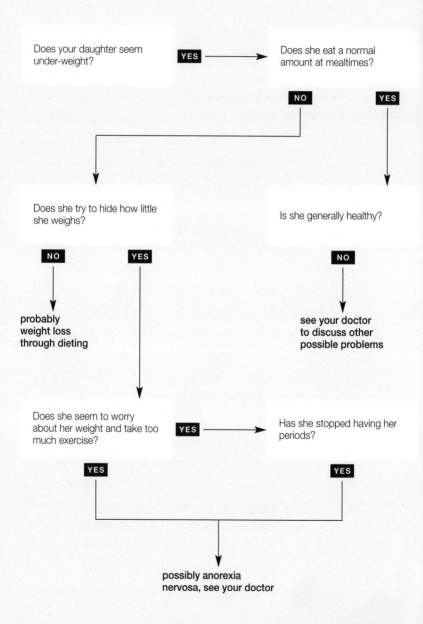

Does your daughter seem under-weight?

YES →

Does she eat a normal amount at mealtimes?

NO

YES

Does she try to hide how little she weighs?

Is she generally healthy?

NO

YES

NO

probably weight loss through dieting

see your doctor to discuss other possible problems

Does she seem to worry about her weight and take too much exercise?

YES →

Has she stopped having her periods?

YES

YES

possibly anorexia nervosa, see your doctor

The results of self-imposed starvation are similar to those of a famine, except that anorexics usually eat adequate amounts of protein and take vitamin tablets. In contrast to the listlessness of those who have starvation forced upon them, anorexics are restless and over-active, especially in the early mornings.

The main physical effects come from the body's attempts to conserve energy. There is weight loss: inessential fat is shed first, followed by muscle, including the heart muscle. The loss of fat does not include the breasts. The monthly periods cease. Body temperature is low, and unlike the normal situation, lowest in the evening. The hands and feet are icy cold, blue or red, and there may be chilblains. Some sufferers have Raynaud's phenomenon of dead-white, numb fingers that are painful to warm up. The blood pressure is low, causing dizziness and frequent fainting. Pulse rate is slow, down to 40–60 beats per minute, but racing in response to food. The skin is dry and, particularly in the younger anorexics, a growth of downy hair, called lanugo (Latin for woolliness) occurs on the face and back. However, head hair does not grow and becomes dry and harsh, although the pubic and under-arm hair remains normal. There is extreme constipation, apart from 'hunger diarrhoea', which consists of small, liquid, greenish motions composed of bile and debris from the intestines. Large amounts of urine are passed, unconnected with how much the girl drinks. There is also nocturia (having to get up to pass water in the night). Swollen ankles and sometimes oedema (fluid accumulating in the tissues) elsewhere also occurs, partly because of the sluggish circulation. Occasionally there are epileptic fits. Psychological effects include anxiety, which the anorexic relates to the fear of eating, and insomnia, with early waking.

45 I know that anorexics and bulimics sometimes abuse laxatives. What effect does that have?

Both anorexics and bulimics may use laxatives excessively, aiming to get rid of their food before it can be absorbed. Anorexics keep obsessionally to routine – including daily laxatives, with an inevitable increase in dosage for them to retain their efficacy. This is more deadly than the irregular way in which bulimics binge and then take a handful of laxatives, but at other times manage to diet. 'Catharticcolon' develops, when the gut no longer responds, however large the dose of laxative.

Laxative abuse may start innocently, to correct the constipation resulting from starvation; often bran is used. This acts not only as a laxative but as a substitute for nourishing food. After finding mild laxatives ineffectual, the anorexic moves on to the stimulants, all of which are basically poisons. They include senna and bisacodyl. The effect is all the more damaging since they are acting on an empty colon. The immediate effect is severe colic, doubling the victim up. The resulting 'motion' mainly comprises water, often blood-stained from the violence of the evacuation, together with mucus and a large amount of protein and vital body minerals, especially potassium.

Hypokalaemia, a low level of potassium in the blood, is a dangerous condition that causes muscular weakness. An early symptom is backache. Later, all the muscles become stiff and feeble, and if the girl has a carbohydrate meal they may become temporarily paralysed. She passes water more often than usual, suffers from constant thirst, but panics when she drinks, because her weight goes up – temporarily. Heart problems may ensue and are potentially serious. There may be mental apathy, poor memory and concentration.

Eighty per cent of anorexics are tempted to take what seems like a short-cut to weight loss – getting rid of the food before the body has actually had any time to absorb it. Bulimia (otherwise known as the bingeing disorder) typically starts with overeating and overweight, and both anorexics and bulimics often use alcohol in order to make it easier for them to vomit.

There are local effects on the hands and teeth. Since self-induced vomiting by putting the fingers down the throat is likely to occur several times a day, the scars of rubbing by the front teeth show up on the back of (usually) the right hand. The acid of the vomit attacks the enamel of the teeth, making them discoloured like those of a 90-year-old. Later, the underlying dentine is also affected, so that the tooth substance is gradually dissolved away.

The general effects are even more harmful than those of laxative abuse. Vital minerals, such as potassium and magnesium, are lost, plus the hydrochloric acid that is unique to the stomach. Potassium shortage causes backache, loss of the knee-jerk reflex and poor mental functioning. Magnesium lack has a direct effect on the nervous system. There may be trembling fits like those of epilepsy, depression, agitation, confusion and even hallucinations. Loss of stomach acid and potassium together cause a toxic condition called alkalosis, in which the blood and all the body fluids are overloaded with alkali, mainly sodium bicarbonate. This may lead to tetany – twitches and spasms of the muscles of the hands, feet and face first, and finally all over. There may also be apathy, altered personality, delirium or stupor. Kidney impairment may cause a build-up of urea in the bloodstream (uraemia) in long-standing cases. There is no effective treatment for potentially life-threatening alkalosis or magnesium lack without first giving up the vomiting.

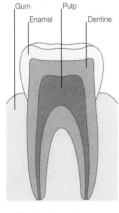

Gum　Pulp
Enamel　Dentine

Self-induced vomiting can damage teeth. The bile and digestive juices which are thrown up act as an acid removing the protective enamel.

47 I read about functional disorders in a magazine. Can you clarify what they are and how they affect the digestive system?

Functional disorders have physical symptoms but the causes are psychological, usually unrecognized by the person concerned. A simple example might be vomiting because of anxiety about your forthcoming marriage, although you insist that you are looking forward to the great day. When it has passed the vomiting is likely to stop soon afterwards. What complicates matters is that the physical symptom, in this case vomiting, may lead to other problems, such as weight loss, or you may have a functional disorder at the same time as an organic one. Dyspepsia may be due to peptic ulcer or to anxiety – and you may have both.

Abdominal pain is a common symptom that may be due to a physical condition such as Crohn's disease or to the common but complex irritable bowel syndrome, which is functional.

Organic pain is usually boring, aching or gripping, whereas functional pain is pricking, stabbing, dramatic ('like a red-hot poker'). Organic pain is usually felt in one place, while functional pain moves around, or is 'all over'. Organic pain fluctuates, and may wake you up; functional pain is often continuous after you wake up. Symptoms that are unlikely to have an organic cause include fullness without overeating, bloating, continuous nausea or burning pain, and belching.

There are certain disorders that are no longer recognized as causes of pain: these include abdominal adhesions after an operation, chronic appendicitis and chronic cholecystitis. There are also some disorders that, while present, may not give rise to pain: these include diverticulosis, hiatus hernia and gallstones. Constipation may have a physical cause, or it may be a symptom of depression. Diarrhoea, similarly, may have a physical cause, or may be due to strong emotions of either revulsion or anxiety. Globus, the feeling of having a lump in the throat (but which does not prevent your swallowing), is a reaction to stress, unlike an organic swallowing difficulty.

What is heartburn, and why do women so often get it during pregnancy? Can I prevent it?

Heartburn, or pyrosis, is an intense burning and sharp, gripping pain in the chest area caused by a reflux (flowing back) from the stomach of acid, pepsin and bile. The mucous membrane which lines your oesophagus, unlike that of the stomach, is not resistant to these digestive chemicals and becomes irritated and inflamed. Faulty muscle contractions in the oesophagus also play a part by being unable to counteract the reflux. You are likely to have a hiatus hernia which increases the reflux, and your mouth may fill with bitter-tasting fluid. The symptoms are worse when you stoop or lie down in bed, or following a large, greasy meal.

Up to 50 per cent of expectant mothers suffer from heartburn up to the time of the birth, but then it stops. The causes are increased pressure on the stomach pushing its contents upwards, from the uterus, plus a hormonal effect, relaxing the lower oesophageal sphincter – the ring of muscle that normally prevents reflux.

In patients who suffer from heartburn a vicious circle of reflux oesophagitis leads to poor clearing of the oesophagus into the stomach, causing incompetence of the sphincter, thus causing more reflux. Some people have a particularly sensitive gullet lining, and alcohol, cigarettes and chocolate all make the sphincter relax.

To try to prevent heartburn, you should reduce any excess weight and avoid constricting clothes. Do not have late or large meals at night. Cut out smoking and avoid alcohol, fruit juice and hot drinks – they irritate the gullet. Avoid taking tablets or capsules at bedtime, but if you must, then have plenty of water. Raise the bedhead 15cm (6ins). You could take an antacid medication, however, these should only be taken if proscribed by your doctor.

Stomach & Abdomen

The stomach and abdomen are the two most obvious sites of digestive disruption and illness. They are responsible for some of the most common afflictions, ranging from indigestion to various types of abdominal pain, as well as being themselves prone to some of the rarest and most serious. It is useful to be able to distinguish between the different ailments and know how to identify their causes in order to give yourself the best chance of preventing and alleviating them. Understanding the way diseases affect your stomach and digestive tract can help you to prevent further complications from arising.

49 What is dyspepsia, and are there different types? Is it the same thing as gastritis?

Dyspepsia or indigestion is pain associated with eating, and felt in the lower chest or upper left-hand side of the abdomen – the epigastrium (meaning that it lies over the stomach). The pain, while it is unpleasant, is not usually extreme. There are two main types, physical and psychological. A common physical cause is alcohol – worse if combined with smoking. Characteristically it occurs in the mornings, with retching (dry heaves), nausea and sometimes vomiting. Peptic ulcer (gastric or duodenal) is partly due to the stomach's own hydrochloric acid attacking its lining membrane, but an underlying problem is infection with the organism helicobacter pylori. Certain drugs, for example many of the most commonly used pain-killers, some steroids, many antibiotics and all the anti-inflammatories, may also cause dyspepsia. There are other less common causes, including cancer of the stomach, disease of the gallbladder and pancreas, disorders of the small intestine, such asulcerative colitis, kidney disease, diabetes and other general system disorders.

The stomach is the mirror of the mind, so psychological factors can cause dyspepsia. Children get 'Monday morning tummy-aches' when they do not want to go to school, and in some adults pain, loss of appetite, nausea and vomiting symbolize their emotions. Indications that the dyspepsia is 'nervous' are varied – fullness, nausea, bloating. There may be dislike of anything touching the abdomen, such as tight clothing, or foods that 'don't agree' with the sufferer. Fatigue, headache and insomnia are often associated with the dyspepsia.

Gastritis is a term often used by lay people to mean dyspepsia. Medically it means something different and more definite – irritation and inflammation of the stomach. Acute gastritis occurs in food-poisoning, but chronic gastritis (common in the elderly) may cause no symptoms. It may sometimes be due to infection with helicobacter pylori, and cause ulcer-type pain.

Q

50 What can I do
to alleviate my
dyspepsia? Can
I prevent it, for
instance if I am
going out for a
special meal?

The best way to alleviate discomfort or pain depends on your type of dyspepsia and its cause. In general, however, there are three quick-fix, temporary solutions. You can take an over-the-counter indigestion medicine; sip a drink of milk slowly; or try a herbal carminative (soothing medicine), of which the best and most widely available is peppermint tea. Commercial tablets are basically alkalis and neutralize the stomach acid, preventing it attacking the stomach lining. These should only be taken as short-term relief.

To prevent dyspepsia on that special occasion, the first essential is to avoid stress during the day. Remember that stress often arises from emotional conflict or badly organized time – so allow enough time to change your mental state, as well as your clothes (wear nothing that constricts you at the waist). Do not be tempted to have an alcoholic drink before you go out – have some milk or cool peppermint tea. Take an antacid tablet that dissolves in your mouth just before you begin eating. Opt for small portions of food and, where there is a choice, go for the simplest dish on offer. Stick to fruit, vegetables, rice, pasta and potatoes whilst avoiding hot curries, rich sauces, creamy sweets and excess black coffee. Be sparing with alcohol, avoid spirits and choose white wines over red.

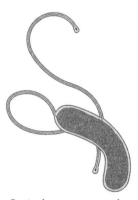

Peptic ulcers are not caused by stress and good living alone, but by the bacteria helicobacter pylori, which is found in the stomach of ulcer sufferers.

51

What is non-ulcer
dyspepsia and how
can I tell it is not a
peptic ulcer?

Non-ulcer dyspepsia means that the symptoms are those of a peptic ulcer but that, however thoroughly the stomach and duodenum are investigated, no ulcer can be found.

Strictly speaking, a peptic ulcer is one that crops up anywhere that stomach acid has eroded the mucous membrane lining the digestive system. Usually it occurs in the stomach or duodenum, and has a propensity to affect men more than women. The main symptom is pain in the epigastrium (high on the left of the abdomen). It is seldom severe, but persists for an hour or so intermittently during the day. The pain is boring, gnawing or burning and you can often point to exactly where it hurts. The pain often occurs when the stomach is empty and is relieved by eating. Immediate relief comes from a dose of antacid, food or drink (not alcohol). Vomiting also stops the pain. Waterbrash and heartburn may occur, and night pain is characteristic, waking you in the small hours, but relieved by a drink and a biscuit.

In non-ulcer dyspepsia the pain often lasts all day, but does not wake you at night. The site of the pain is often diffuse and variable. Women are affected twice as often as men. Some foods make the symptoms worse and antacids do not always help. Vomiting does not relieve the pain. You feel 'out of sorts', with a headache, lack of energy and poor sleep.

Q

52 I have non-ulcer
dyspepsia. What
is the treatment
likely to be?

If you have non-ulcer dyspepsia, with the symptoms of peptic ulcer, the first essential is to make sure that there really is no ulcer. Your symptoms and an ordinary examination are not enough. Special investigations are needed. These may include a barium meal, in which you swallow a glass of thick, white liquid containing barium. This shows up on an x-ray, outlining the stomach and duodenum. It may show an ulcer crater or a tell-tale deformity of the duodenum from scarring, but 20 per cent of results are false negatives – an ulcer fails to show. Or you might have an endoscopy: this is more accurate and has the advantage that a biopsy (sample of tissue) may be taken for checking under the microscope. An endoscope (in this case a gastroscope) is a flexible fibre-optic tube that is passed into the stomach, allowing the operator to see inside it and the duodenum. Alternatively, a urease breath test is done to check for infection with helicobacter pylori, a bacterium that makes the stomach lining less able to resist acid. If the test for helicobacter pylori is positive you need a course of antibiotics and checks in the future that the infection has not recurred; antacids may also help. And you should review possible causes of stress during the last six months. This may mean a change in lifestyle. Improvement of your general health may also help.

I often suffer from painful indigestion and sometimes other symptoms during or after meals. Which foods should I eat and which should I avoid to prevent this happening?

Unless you sit over your meals for hours, not many foods give you symptoms right away unless they are too hot, too cold or excessively spicy. An immediate reaction – including swelling lips, vomiting and a runny nose – can only be due to allergy. You can become allergic to almost any food, but the most common offenders are cow's milk, eggs, wheat, soya, peanuts and shellfish.

To avoid strain on your digestive system, cut out alcohol, strong tea and coffee; anything fried; gravies and soups made with meat extracts; raw vegetables; raw, unripe fruit; pips and skin of all fruit (including cooked or in jam); dried fruit; pickles, spices and condiments; tough, twice-cooked, or highly seasoned meat; fatty fish (salmon, sardines); rich puddings; new bread and hot buttered toast; rye or wheat crispbread; cakes containing fruit, nuts or peel.

Foods to choose include weak tea or coffee; milk, yoghurt, cottage cheese, eggs; white fish (steamed, baked or boiled); chicken, lean ham, tender beef or lamb; crisp toast (buttered, cold); white bread; plain biscuits (Marie); honey, golden syrup, jelly; cornflour, semolina, ground rice, oatflour porridge; junket, jelly, custard, blancmange; potatoes (boiled or baked, no skin); cooked, puréed green or yellow vegetables; stewed fruit (baked apple); purées, fruit fools; fruit juices (strained and diluted).

A lot of my middle-
aged friends have a
hiatus hernia. What
exactly is this, and
how can I avoid it?

Normally, a ring of muscle at the junction of the gullet and the stomach (the gastro-oesophageal sphincter) prevents the stomach contents going back up the oesophagus. This tends to slacken from around 50-plus and pressure from the abdomen can cause a hiatus hernia, a bulge of stomach pushing up into the chest. There are three types: sliding, para-oesophageal and mixed (see illustration). The symptoms are heartburn if you stoop or lie down; regurgitation of your food; swallowing discomfort, with a feeling like a lump in the chest; pain behind the breastbone when you eat; and 'wind'.

To avoid hiatus hernia you should exercise, because all your muscles tighten up, including the sphincter. Maintain an upright posture and check any excess weight. Avoid making a strong physical effort and bending down at the same time: use long-handled tools for gardening or housework. Do not wear tight belts or eat large meals in the evening, or chocolate – it relaxes the sphincter. Raise the head of your bed a few inches. Use alkaline medicines after meals if you get heartburn. Ask your pharmicist about medication which speeds up the emptying of the oesophagus. Use a linctus if you have a cough. Eat plenty of fruit and vegetables and avoid straining when you pass a motion.

*A hiatus hernia is a small
envelope of the stomach
protruding through the
diaphragm which causes
pain in the upper section
of the abdomen.*

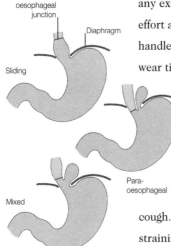

Gastro-
oesophageal
junction

Diaphragm

Sliding

Para-
oesophageal

Mixed

I suffer from 'wind'
and find it both
uncomfortable and
embarrassing. Where
does it come from
and what can I do
about it?

'Wind' can go in two directions – up, leading to belching and down. They are both uncomfortable but wind from the back passage (flatus) is the more embarrassing.

In belching, the wind consists entirely of air you have swallowed, often gulping it down with a long drink. Babies and beer drinkers are notorious for this. Flatus, the more troublesome wind from the back passage, also comes largely from swallowed air, passing through the tortuous tubing of the digestive system. On its way, the oxygen is absorbed so that what remains is mainly nitrogen.

There are two other sources for wind below. A chemical interaction between bicarbonate from your food and the hydrochloric acid in your stomach may release carbon dioxide. Bacterial fermentation occurring in the large intestine produces carbon dioxide, hydrogen and methane. It is methane in the stools that makes them float. The total gas in the digestive system at any time is around 200 ml, but wind is often associated with bloating, when it feels like much more. Sometimes you may be taking a medicine that boosts gas production in the gut.

To reduce these symptoms, practise not taking down air every time you swallow, and do your drinking and eating with your mouth closed. Since anxiety increases your propensity for swallowing air, sort out any worries through discussion and perhaps by taking a small dose of a tranquillizer. Cut out any medication you do not really need. Trouble-makers include the common antibiotics, ask your pharmicist for their advice if you are unsure about any medication you are on, and for advice to help treat the condition. Modify your diet by omitting beans, other legumes and the cabbage family and by restricting your fibre intake – from fruits, fresh or dried, bran cereals and wholemeal flour. Drink separately from eating.

56

I have a bitter-tasting fluid that sometimes fills my mouth. My doctor says it is waterbrash. What is this and where does it come from?

The fluid that spontaneously fills your mouth is likely to be from more than one source. Simple waterbrash consists of only the watery type of saliva that is produced by the parotid glands – those involved in mumps. Normally you produce about a litre of saliva every day. The overproduction of watery saliva is called ptyalism, which generally occurs as a reaction to irritation in the mouth. Waterbrash is a particular type of ptyalism, but in this case the trigger is irritation of the stomach from bad food, a peptic ulcer or an emotional shock that 'makes you feel sick'. The salivary glands begin making saliva at 20 times their usual rate, in bursts or paroxysms – and you are suddenly aware of your mouth being full of fluid. The purpose of the extra fluid is to dilute and help wash away something from the upper part of your digestive system that has irritated your stomach. On the same principle, it is common to have a smaller increase in the flow of saliva when you are about to vomit.

While saliva is tasteless, the juices made by the stomach are acid, and bile produced by the liver is bitter. Bile enters the digestive system in the duodenum, the first few inches of intestine, and is mixed with the stomach's contents – particularly in any stomach upset. There are several reasons (apart from vomiting) for some of the stomach contents rising into your mouth. These include simple regurgitation, especially after a big meal or one that included a lot of liquid, a reflux leakage back upwards of the stomach's contents or a hiatus hernia. The regurgitation occurs spontaneously, but not with the suddenness of waterbrash. In your case you have waterbrash that is mixed with material from your stomach, giving it a bitter taste.

It is not uncommon to feel sick, have a stomach upset or even vomit after a fatty meal. This is not due to allergy, but you may have a sensitivity to fats, which can apply to any food, without identifiable reason. Children (and adults) who will not eat fat on meat are in this group. Fat takes longer to digest than carbohydrates and proteins.

After passing through the mouth and the stomach, where it is bathed in digestive enzymes and hydrochloric acid, fat is virtually unchanged. It is only when it reaches the duodenum that the digestion of fat can actually begin. Digestive enzymes made in the pancreas, and bile that is manufactured by the liver, are both poured onto the part-digested food in the intestine, in response to an electro-chemical signal that fatty food is on its way. Lipase from the pancreas then emulsifies the fats, breaking down the fat globules into smaller ones. Bile completes this process.

It is only when the globules are microscopically small that they can be absorbed into the bloodstream. If this does not happen, fatty diarrhoea results – the motions are pale and full of undigested fat called steatorrhoea. Pancreatic or liver disease (for instance, pancreatitis, hepatitis or cirrhosis) will prevent the digestion and absorption of fats – but you will still feel very ill.

Gallstones do not cause an intolerance to fatty food. The dyspeptic and vague general symptons that are often ascribed to gallstones are more likely to be due to an irritable colon, diverticular disease, a peptic ulcer or to simple dyspepsia. Gallstones usually cause no symptons, unless they are what is known as 'impacted'.

If you have discomfort when you eat fats it is, however, sensible to cut down on them – particularly eggs, chocolate, cheese and nuts.

58 What causes
gallstones and what
are the symptons?

Gallstones are of two types: made from cholesterol and pigment. Cholesterol stones are far more common in Western cultures and can arise due to several factors: an excess of cholesterol in the bile (cholesterolosis), due to eating too much; an excess of mucin, the slimy material that protects the gallbladder from bile salts; a condition known as 'the stagnant pool' – a sluggish flow of bile so that the gallbladder does not empty properly; or an overworking of the gallbladder, so that cholesterol crystallizes out to form stones. Pigment stones are due to exessive concentration of bile and calcium in the gallbladder, or to a liver disorder.

There are some predisposing factors that make you more likely to produce gallstones. These include taking extra oestrogen from the contraceptive pill, hormone therapy or having borne several children; being overweight; taking tranquillizing medicines; eating small, fat-free meals; or being over 40. By the age of 40, 20 per cent of us have gallstones, but they only cause symptoms if they get wedged in one of the bile ducts. The effect that should alert you is pain. Biliary colic is mild to agonizing continuous pain, felt in the upper right-hand quadrant of the abdomen and between the shoulder blades or at the tip of the right shoulder. Cholecystitis (inflammation of the gallbladder) also causes pain.

What is the medical treatment for gallstones and what can I do to help myself?

Gallstones that are not causing symptoms are best left undisturbed, but if you have had one attack of biliary colic from an impacted stone, you are at considerable risk of further attacks. Treatment may not involve an operation, for your doctor could prescribe bile acid treatment. The principle is to dissolve the cholesterol of the stones with medicine that specifically dilutes the bile. They must be pure cholesterol stones, not too many, none more than 15mm in diameter, and the gallbladder must be emptying effectively. The medication is a mixture of bile acids in capsules, taken once a day, at bedtime. The disadvantages of this method are that it takes 18 months plus to work, during which time you must not risk pregnancy, you may have pain during treatment and the stones often recur later. Rowachol treatment involves using six chemicals – monoturpines – dissolved in olive oil, which are taken nightly, also for 18 months. These work by preventing the formation of cholesterol crystals. Direct-contact dissolution involves a liquid containing a chemical that dissolves cholesterol; it is injected through a long needle directly into the gallbladder, and you have a sedative or anaesthetic for the procedure. It does not matter how big or how many stones there

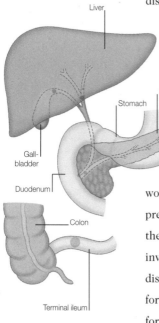

Liver

Pancreas

Stomach

Gall-
bladder

Duodenum

Colon

Terminal ileum

Gallstones are hard lumps, shown here by the small shaded areas, that vary in size up to that of a pea. These stop the gallbladder from working properly and cause pain.

are. And in shock-wave lithotripsy the gallstones are shattered by focusing sound waves on them through the skin. The fragments are then easily dissolved in bile acid treatment and washed away in the bile. The whole process is painless and takes half an hour. However, despite all the above, surgery remains the best option in difficult cases.

If you want to help yourself the best things to do are to correct any overweight problem – gradually. Avoid refined white sugar, for instance in soft drinks; do not smoke; and eat other vegetables than legumes. The good news is that alcohol and coffee in moderation are acceptable.

60 I'm told that acute cholecystitis is inflammation of the gallbladder, similar to acute appendicitis. Is this true and what are the symptoms?

Acute cholecystitis, inflammation of the gallbladder, is almost always caused by a stone blocking its duct, much as appendicitis can be caused by a nut or other debris getting lodged in the appendix. The inflammation goes through two phases: chemical irritation from bile salts trapped in the gallbladder is followed by bacterial infection in the stagnant bile.

The symptoms worsen from one phase to the next. The cardinal symptom is pain. Although it is called colic, the pain does not come in spasms (as in green-apple colic), but is continuous, varying in intensity from mild to very severe. Restlessness occurs due to the severity of the pain. There may be vomiting, sweating, pallor, a moist skin and high fever, sometimes accompanied by rigors. These are attacks of shivering in which you feel deadly cold, although you are actually burning hot, with a very high temperature. Your pulse is racing (something that your doctor will easily detect), while you may feel your heart thumping quickly.

Guarding is a reflex to protect the gallbladder: at the lightest touch you feel the muscles of the right upper quadrant of your abdomen tense up. Murphy's sign is a similar protective reflex, in which your abdominal muscles involuntarily pull tight when you breathe in. There will be tenderness at the smallest pressure in the gallbladder area, with swelling of the tissues in this part, due to fluid. It 'gives' to make a little pit if you press it with your finger – just like ankle oedema. Jaundice is another symptom: a general yellowing of your tissues, most noticeable in the whites of your eyes and your skin.

61 How will I be treated for acute cholecystitis?

The chances are that your acute cholecystitis will wake you in the middle of the night with severe abdominal pain, so that you call the doctor in straight away. He will probably send you to hospital via the Accident and Emergency Department – all the more urgently if you are in a vulnerable group (say, diabetic or over 70).

The ideal is for treatment to be set in train before the infection has become established. Very occasionally the acute inflammation will subside spontaneously, but this is a trap. It is highly dangerous to delay treatment – you stand a substantial risk of empyema, when the gallbladder is one big abscess, or a stone may break through its wall spilling pus and bacteria, causing life-threatening peritonitis. Cholecystectomy, the surgical removal of the gallbladder, is the only effective treatment. It is a safe, long-established operation. There are three versions: the standard is incisional. It involves a cut large enough for the surgeon to examine all round the abdomen, using normal-sized instruments. In the mini-incisional type the cut is much smaller, heals more quickly and leaves a smaller scar. Laparoscopic (keyhole or minimal-access) surgery is modern, fashionable and needs an even shorter recovery time. It requires a specially trained surgeon in a major centre, as the operation is delicate, and there is more risk of some complication being missed. You are off work for an average of 5–12 weeks, 34 days or 7 days respectively after each of these operations.

If you are weak and the surgeon doesn't want to put you through the strains of a major operation, he may prefer to do a cholecystostomy. This means making a small hole in the gallbladder to let out the pus and remove any stone – then sewing up. You can then have the full operation when you are stronger.

62 What should I do
if a member of my
family gets severe
abdominal pain?

Any severe pain in the abdomen demands serious concern. It is a warning of potential disaster. The victim cannot help himself or herself, so the responsibility falls on you. You must reassure your relative that all will be well and that you will get the necessary help. Keep repeating soothing words. Leave him the way he feels most comfortable, and give him a hot-water bottle or heated pad to hold against his abdomen. Call the doctor urgently. If you are really worried, call for an emergency ambulance. Organize your thoughts so that you can give the facts clearly and succinctly to the practice nurse, the doctor or the hospital. It will help them to assess the situation and they will take you more seriously.

There are a number of questions you may need to answer. Where is the pain? Did it come on suddenly, or build up over several hours? Did it start at a precise time, which would indicate something like a perforation? Has he had similar, but perhaps less severe, attacks before? Does he suffer from indigestion? Has he complained of his stomach swelling up? Is he on any medication? Has he had any other health problems in the last six months? Has he had any chest or heart problems? Has he vomited? Has he got diarrhoea? Is he short of breath? If the patient is a woman, could she be pregnant? Does she have any period problems?

The common causes of severe abdominal pain fall into two groups: those coming on suddenly (for example, perforation of the gallbladder or haemorrhage from an ulcer or cancer) and those that build up more gradually. In the more gradual group we can distinguish pain due to inflammation or infection – names ending in '-itis'; pain due to blockage of a duct or of the intestine; and various medical disorders.

Acute appendicitis is inflammation in this small, blind end of the gut (the size of your little finger), coming off the first part of the large bowel and lying in the bottom right-hand corner of the abdomen. Acute cholecystitis is inflammation affecting the gallbladder, in the opposite corner of the abdomen – top centre and left. Biliary colic is due to blockage by a gallstone of the gallbladder or one of the bile ducts; perforated (burst) peptic ulcers may be gastric, duodenal or in the oesophagus; obstruction of the gut is often due to a strangulated hernia; and peritonitis is inflammation of the membrane that encloses the abdominal organs, secondarily to infection in one of them.

Non-specific pain is acute abdominal pain that remains undiagnosed, even if a laparotomy – an operation to look inside the abdomen – is performed. These cases do not develop, at any rate not on this occasion. Some may be due to irritable colon, others to trapped wind. There are also some occasional causes of acute abdominal pain. Acute pancreatitis is often due to long-established alcohol excess, but not invariably so. Diverticulitis is due to acute inflammation of one or more diverticula. Cancer of the stomach or the colon may cause pain, and so may a blood clot blocking a vessel to part of the gut. An aneurysm of the aorta, the main artery running down the middle of the body, is yet another cause of pain. The medical causes of pain include diabetes, shingles, pleurisy and heart attack.

The type of abdominal pain from which you are suffering provides vital clues to the underlying problem. Visceral pain comes directly from the internal organs (the viscera) and is caused only by distension. It is localized vaguely to 'somewhere in the abdomen'. Somatic pain, by contrast, is due to inflammation of the membrane covering the affected organ and is felt in a very particular location. Diverticular disease, for example, produces pain and tenderness in the left lower quadrant of the abdomen.

Duodenal ulcer pain is characteristically burning or gnawing. Intestinal obstruction causes cramp-like pains, while intestinal angina is felt as intense, steady and crushing pain round the navel (it is relieved by the same drugs as angina in the chest).

Biliary colic is continuous pain but it is not in fact colicky. Pain that is related to a woman's periods is usually due to endometriosis, pelvic inflammatory disease, degeneration of a fibroid or salpingitis (which is an infection in the fallopian tubes).

Colic occurs in cycles of pain, building to a crescendo and then subsiding to nothing, over and over again. Colic due to disease of the colon has a slow cycle, while a shorter cycle and intense pain comes from renal colic – in kidney disease. Colic from the small intestine cycles twice as fast; and gallstone colic produces the most rapid cycle of all, with high-intensity pain throughout which subsides dramatically if the stone shifts position.

Peritonitis causes non-stop pain, which worsens if you so much as move a muscle, but after a while returns to its previous intensity. A peptic ulcer gives less severe pain, increasing periodically for an hour or so at a time.

Diagnosing digestive problems is often aided by the areas in which pain is felt. In this illustration the abdomen is divided into a grid, pain in each section corresponds to a particular disorder.

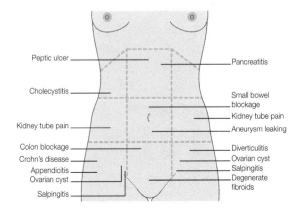

Peptic ulcer

Cholecystitis

Kidney tube pain

Colon blockage

Crohn's disease

Appendicitis

Ovarian cyst

Salpingitis

Pancreatitis

Small bowel blockage

Kidney tube pain

Aneurysm leaking

Diverticulitis

Ovarian cyst

Salpingitis

Degenerate fibroids

65 What causes long-
term abdominal
pain? Can you give
me a checklist of
signs that I should
look out for?

Up to 50 per cent of those attending a gastroenterological ('tum and guts') clinic are there because of chronic abdominal pain, which is defined as pain that continues for more than three months. It is often functional, and no definite physical cause is found in three times as many cases as are diagnosed with peptic ulcer and oesophagitis.

Certain common disorders cause long-term pain. In the stomach area there is peptic ulcer (including gastric, duodenal and oesophageal), stomach cancer and nervous dyspepsia. Related to the colon is diverticular disease, inflammatory bowel disorders (ulcerative colitis, Crohn's disease), irritable bowel syndrome, constipation and cancer of the colon.

There are certain signs to watch out for. Pain, vomiting and diarrhoea force themselves on your attention. Less obvious are loss of body hair, appetite or weight, without dieting; 'liverpalms' (the palms of the hands becoming warm and red); unaccustomed constipation or chronic diarrhoea; any recent change in bowel routine; the abdomen getting bigger without the body becoming fatter; discomfort after eating particular foods; loud borborygmi (stomach gurgles); passing motions of an unusual colour or with mucus; a sensation of something sticking when you swallow or of food coming back into your mouth spontaneously; and hunger pains.

There is a well-worn pathway of symptoms in acute appendicitis, which over half of sufferers experience over 24 hours. The pain starts with colicky pain round the navel, changing after a few hours to a relentless pain in the right, lower corner of your abdomen. An ordinary stomach upset usually hurts in the epigastrium (the middle to left of the upper third of your abdomen), and the pain is colicky, but does not change in character or position.

Loss of appetite occurs in appendicitis and you may vomit once, but no more. In a stomach upset nausea and vomiting are likely to persist, at least for a few hours. In appendicitis you feel definitely ill; but you feel 'well in yourself' with a stomach upset. The mode of onset also differs. While appendicitis comes out of the blue and there is obvious cause, a stomach upset may be due to infectious gastroenteritis or to eating something that disagrees with you. Someone with appendicitis will look flushed and have a slightly raised temperature – not more than 38.3°C (100.9°F). If a stomach upset is an infective sort, the victim may have a raised temperature, but feels cold and clammy. If you do nothing (a dangerous decision if you suspect appendicitis) the right-sided pain will worsen as peritonitis sets in. With a stomach upset you may have some diarrhoea, but the illness is likely to leave you within 48 hours.

APPENDICITIS/STOMACH UPSET

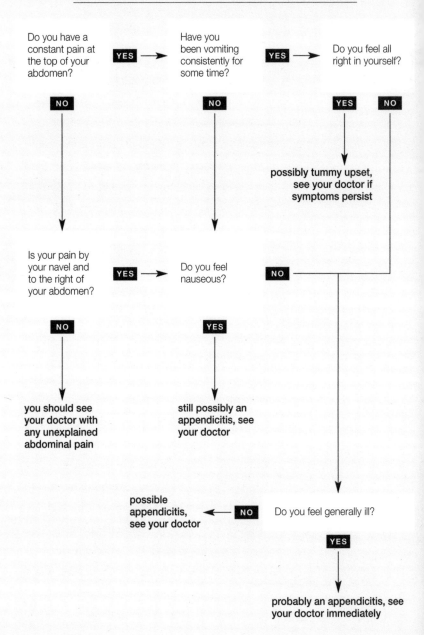

Do you have a constant pain at the top of your abdomen?

YES →

Have you been vomiting consistently for some time?

YES →

Do you feel all right in yourself?

NO

NO

YES **NO**

possibly tummy upset, see your doctor if symptoms persist

Is your pain by your navel and to the right of your abdomen?

YES →

Do you feel nauseous?

NO

NO

YES

you should see your doctor with any unexplained abdominal pain

still possibly an appendicitis, see your doctor

possible appendicitis, see your doctor

← **NO**

Do you feel generally ill?

YES

probably an appendicitis, see your doctor immediately

The symptoms that should alert you to problems with your colon are pain, diarrhoea, constipation, distension and blood in the motions. Pain from the colon is felt below the navel, either in the middle or on the left. A host of disorders, both acute and chronic, can cause it – ranging from food poisoning to Crohn's disease. Diarrhoea implies motions that are too loose and too frequent. It may be acute, as in a case of gastroenteritis that is due to such organisms as salmonella or campylobacter. Chronic diarrhoea occurs in inflammatory bowel disease, overactive thyroid, or as a result of too much alcohol.

Simple constipation may be due to a diet that is short in fibre and may just cause discomfort, but constipation that comes on rapidly may be due to cancer – although irritable bowel syndrome is a more likely cause. Distension is commonly due to the colonic muscles getting out of synchrony, but excessive gas production may result from too much fibre (especially beans). It may also signal serious obstruction. Blood in your motions, apart from piles, is likely to come from polyps, cancer or diverticular disease.

Pain in an appendicitis occurs in two stages. At first the pain occurs around the navel area, then moves so it is situated directly over the appendix itself.

First stage

Second stage

My child is thought
to be suffering from
'abdominal migraine',
with recurring bouts
of abdominal pain.
What is the cause
and how should I
treat it?

Every child gets abdominal pain at times and some of them may vomit. Pain recurring over a period of months or years is not uncommon – it affects 15 per cent of children by the age of seven, after this abdominal pain tends to be replaced by migraine headaches. 'Abdominal migraine' covers both, but the term 'Periodic Syndrome' is also used, to include vomiting. The three symptoms may occur together or separately at different times. However, they keep coming back, with or without a trigger, but not necessarily on a regular basis.

A typical attack comes on in the morning. It comprises colicky pain in the middle of the abdomen, and the child looks pale and wants to lie down. He or she may vomit, and in some this is the chief symptom. If investigations have not come up with a physical cause, it is counterproductive to repeat them. It is now time to look at the child's personality and the emotional background. Susceptible children are usually intelligent and tend to be tense, fussy, anxious and over-conscientious. They are poor mixers and often had an early background of nightmares, bed-wetting and finicky eating. Management of the problem is based on discussion and explanation, support and encouragement with a qualified specialist child therapist.

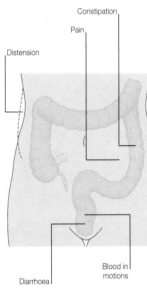

Constipation

Pain

Distension

Blood in
motions

Diarrhoea

*Abdominal migraine
is comprised of several
symptoms including pain,
distension of the abdominal
area and problems with
the motions.*

Referred pain is felt in a particular area of the skin, although the cause originates in a different place, usually an internal organ like the liver, stomach or colon. A well-known example is pain from coronary artery disease of the heart producing pain in the left arm and the jaw. Similarly, pain from an inflamed gallbladder sets off pain in the right shoulder and near the tip of the shoulder blade.

The explanation is that nerve fibres carrying the message about pain share a junction box (or synapse) with nerves coming from other areas of skin. The information relayed onwards in the spinal cord to the brain, where we become conscious of it, combines the input from both sets of fibres.

All the internal organs (a large proportion of which belong to the digestive system) produce referred pain associated with each viscus (internal organ). Pain from a viscus (visceral pain) is more basic than pain felt through the skin or a membrane (somatic or parietal pain). In the case of acute appendicitis it is visceral pain that is felt first.

The oesophagus refers pain to a large area on the left side of your chest; the stomach to a hook-shaped area near the midline; the liver and gallbladder to a place by the tip of the shoulder blade; the colon to a point below the navel, but not as far down as in non-referred pain from other causes.

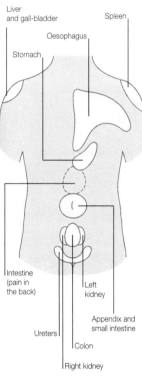

Liver and gall-bladder
Spleen
Oesophagus
Stomach
Intestine (pain in the back)
Left kidney
Ureters
Appendix and small intestine
Colon
Right kidney

The shaded sections in the diagram above show where referred pain is felt, and the underlying problem areas.

Ulcers & Excretion

Ulcers are a common source of confusion, partly because they can occur in various regions of the digestive system and partly because of the variety of names given to them. This section aims to clear up some of the confusion. The health of the bowels is intricately linked to what we eat – many excretory ailments can be remedied simply by a change in diet. The answers given here will help sufferers of bowel problems, including irritable bowel syndrome and diverticular disease, and give advice to those who wish to avoid it.

70 My aunt, aged 65, has just been told she has a peptic ulcer. I thought this only affected stressed businessmen, so why are more and more elderly women getting it nowadays?

For most of the 20th century a peptic ulcer, particularly a duodenal ulcer, was very much a man's illness, especially in those aged 20–50. Even now it affects ten per cent of men at some time, but the figures have turned upside down – it is elderly women who are now suffering something like an epidemic of peptic ulcers, including raised mortality figures. In the 1970s the modern diet was blamed – quick and easy ready meals of carbohydrate and fat, with a lack of vegetable matter and fruit, which become alkaline in the stomach. Executive stress was another favourite 'cause', since men were the chief victims. Since then women have caught up in the importance and stressfulness of their work, and the executive stress explanation no longer holds water. Heredity is a factor, but this applies mostly to those who get their ulcer young – when they are around 20. Lack of resistance by the mucosa (the mucous membrane lining the digestive system) to the damaging effects of the hydrochloric acid and pepsin in our gastric juices also plays a part, as does increased production of acid by the stomach: this increase is measurable in people with ulcers. Another factor is lack of female hormones: these apparently improve the resistance of the mucosa to gastric fluid, so that men, and women past their menopause, are most vulnerable to ulceration. Peptic ulcers in men benefit from taking female hormones, although these can produce feminizing side-effects.

Helicobacter pylori is a germ that attracted attention in the early 1990s, and has been found living just under the mucosa in 90 per cent of those with duodenal ulcers and 60 per cent with gastric ulcers. It is a major cause of the disease.

None of these causes of peptic ulcers accounts for the huge rise in numbers in a particular age and sex group that has occurred recently. It is also this group, senior females, who succumb to the painful condition of arthritis. The medication that helps arthritis sufferers most are the NSAIDs (non-steroidal anti-inflammatory drugs) and it is also these which penetrate the protective layer of mucus covering the mucosa, leaving the stomach wall exposed to the effects of the gastric juices.

71 Can you explain the difference between a peptic ulcer, a gastric ulcer and a duodenal ulcer?

The term 'peptic ulcer' means any ulcer – an eating away of the surface of skin or membrane – in an area where it is exposed to the digestive juices of the stomach, specifically pepsin and hydrochloric acid. The causes of peptic ulcer, wherever it may be, are a high concentration of acid, a high level of pepsin, poor production of mucus, which is alkaline and protects the mucous membrane (mucosa), a poor blood supply that impairs the healthy resistance of the mucosa, and infection with helicobacter pylori.

Gastric ulcers occur in the stomach itself. There may not be an excess of acid with this type, but the mucosal resistance may be reduced by drugs like aspirin. Gastric ulcers are important because of a propensity for them to be cancerous. Duodenal ulcers occur in the duodenum, the 25cm (9in) stretch of intestine that adjoins the stomach; they are the most common type. Oesophageal ulcers are also common, since reflux often occurs, carrying the digestive juices with it. Hiatal ulcers can develop in a hiatus hernia, a pouch of stomach that has slipped up through the ring of muscle at the entrance of the stomach. Diverticular ulcers can develop in a Meckel's diverticulum, a developmental vestige. And marginal ulcers arise following surgery, for instance around a colostomy opening.

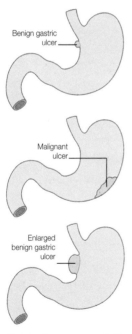

Benign gastric ulcer

Malignant ulcer

Enlarged benign gastric ulcer

Gastric ulcers can occur both within the stomach as well as outside it and may cause the infected areas to become extended.

One treatment for peptic ulcer is the reduction of stressful situations, since anxiety and anger both lead to an increase in acid production in the stomach. Being calm, even sad, can inhibit acid production and increase the flow of mucus, which protects the mucosa (lining of the stomach and oesophagus), and is alkaline. Also, eat small, regular meals and do not smoke.

Antacids, taken three to four times daily and at bedtime, will help with the pain, but something stronger is needed for healing of the ulcer to take place. Hydrogen-receptor antagonists, which reduce the amount of gastric juice (especially the acid), are useful for this purpose. Proton pump inhibitors prevent the final stages of acid production and work more rapidly than the hydrogen-receptor antagonists, and the actual healing of the ulcer is quicker. Hydrogen-receptor antagonists seldom have any side-effects. The proton pump inhibitors, however, may interact with other drugs and cause side-effects such as headaches, and dizziness.

Bismuth salts promote ulcer healing by providing a coating over the base of the ulcer. They also stimulate mucus production and eliminate helicobacter infection. As for drugs that you can buy over the counter, only antacids and bismuth salts are available without prescription. What your doctor is

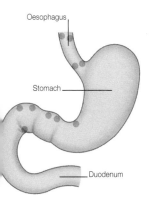

Oesophagus

Stomach

Duodenum

Peptic ulcers are not confined to the stomach but can appear both in the lower oesophagus and the upper duodenum as shown here.

likely to prescribe is 'Triple therapy', which actually comprises a drug to suppress acid production, plus antibiotics to clear the helicobacter infection. There is a 90 per cent success rate for treating duodenal ulcer using this treatment, and a 60 per cent success rate for gastric ulcer.

73 I've just learned that I have a duodenal ulcer. What is the duodenum, and why does it get ulcers?

The duodenum occupies a key position in the digestive system, linking the upper part of mouth, gullet and stomach with the bowels. It also has a key role in the digestive process, as food arriving from the stomach is only half-digested. This applies to starches and fats in particular, but proteins are also incompletely digested.

The word duodenum means '12 fingers' breadth', which is its length. It lies just above the navel, in a circle hugging the head of the pancreas, and is also in close contact with the gallbladder. Its functions involve both these organs. The gallbladder stores bile that has been made in the liver, and empties itself almost completely when it gets the message that food is arriving from the stomach. Between meals, it only lets out a dribble of bile. The bile travels down the bile duct to the duodenum. The pancreatic duct meets it there in the ampulla of Vater, which opens into the duodenum about 8cm (3in) from the stomach. It is guarded by a ring of muscle, or sphincter, controlling the release of bile and

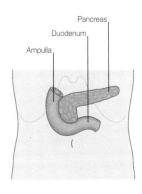

Pancreas
Duodenum
Ampulla

The duodenum has to cope with bile and pancreatic fluid which occasionally irritate the inner lining thus causing ulceration.

pancreatic fluid. Essential digestion takes place in the duodenum. First, bile acts on the fats in the food, breaking them down, then pancreatic enzymes complete the digestion of the remaining starches, fats and proteins. The mucous membrane lining the duodenum has a generous blood supply and is very thick. It contains the duodenal glands. Their secretion neutralizes the acidity of the stomach contents, and contains mucin to protect the mucosa, plus an enzyme to help digest protein.

It is hardly surprising that the duodenum is such a prime site for ulceration, since it has to contend with the acidity of the stomach acids, concentrated bile salts, and the powerful pancreatic enzyme for digesting protein.

74 What herbal remedies are there for dyspepsia and peptic ulcers?

There is a wide choice of herbal remedies for digestive problems. For simple dyspepsia or indigestion the most effective include German chamomile, cardamom, galangal, peppermint, gentian and ginger. They are available as tablets or capsules from most health stores. Of particular value against acidity is a combination of meadowsweet and marshmallow root. Helpful foods include slippery elm gruel, especially at bedtime, mashed bananas and honey. Instead of ordinary tea and coffee after meals, try agrimony, dandelion and chamomile in equal parts, meadowsweet, hops or balm.

For peptic ulcers (gastric or duodenal) the *British Herbal Pharmacopoeia* recommends marshmallow root, dried marigold petals *(Calendula)*, American cranesbill (plant or root), comfrey leaves and liquorice. These are available as tablets, powders, capsules or liquid extracts, with instructions concerning dosage. For drinks, try comfrey, yarrow and meadowsweet, in equal parts; also spring water; carrot, raw white cabbage and other vegetable juices; and potato water, made by boiling potatoes for 20 minutes. For sustaining the nerves drink the juices of lime flowers, skullcap, chamomile or valerian.

You can buy Frank Roberts's complete treatment over the counter. It consists of liquid extracts of goldenseal, poke root, echinacea, American cranesbill, and marshmallow root, 99g (3½oz) of each. Store out of the light and take 15–30 drops three times a day, between meals, for four months.

Herbalists advise having three meals a day, none of them in the late evening. These should be low-fibre, low-fat, low-protein meals, with no added salt; basically a lacto-vegetarian diet – that is, vegetarian but allowing some dairy products. No spicy foods or very hot foods (in either sense) should be eaten, and nothing should be drunk with meals. Dried or mashed banana is good, slippery elm gruel, skimmed cow's milk, soya milk and honey are all acceptable. Vitamin supplements should contain vitamins A, the B-complex vitamins, C, E and K, iron and bromelain (pineapple stem).

75 Will I need surgery
for a peptic ulcer,
and what is the
procedure?

Most people with a peptic ulcer, either gastric or duodenal, will not have to resort to surgery because ulcer-healing drugs are now so effective. However, certain complications force the choice of surgery. Perforation, affecting five per cent of ulcer victims, allows the stomach contents to leak into the peritoneal space causing immediate severe pain, vomiting and shock. This is an emergency and you will be hurried off to the operating theatre immediately. The operation may involve the over-sewing of the place that broke down or cutting out of the affected part. Haemorrhage can occur in 15 per cent of the operations performed. The ulcer extends into one of the larger blood vessels, leading to vomiting of blood, melaena (blood in the motions) or anaemia, found to be due to blood oozing from a particular site. All these require surgical repair. Malignant ulcer, usually the gastric type, also calls for prompt surgery. The outlook is excellent – 95 per cent successful – if the disease is caught very early and the ulcer and surrounding tissue cut away.

Elective operations are necessary if an ulcer relapses despite several courses of ulcer-healing drugs, especially if you have a history of ulcers in your family. A previous episode of perforation or haemorrhage of your ulcer or scarring after ulceration causing either a so-called hour-glass stomach with a constriction round the middle will mean an elective operation is performed..

The procedures that may be used are vagotomy (cutting the nerves that trigger acid production), partial gastrectomy (removal of the ulcer-bearing part of the stomach), gastroenterostomy (forming a shortcut, bypassing much of the duodenum) and pyloroplasty (refashioning the outlet from the stomach to deal with obstruction).

76 What complications might affect me after a stomach operation?

Most people feel very much better and have no further trouble from their digestive system after a stomach operation, but you have a one in six chance of unwanted symptoms. If you have lost a part of the organ you may feel uncomfortably full before the end of the meal. Your stomach will adjust in time, but you must eat little and often. After eating hot, sweet food in particular, you feel over-full, nauseated, faint and weary and drowsy. This is called dumping syndrome. You may also have palpitations and flushes but oddly, the symptoms seem only to happen when you are upright. Small, dry meals with drinks separately, and lying down all help, but you will improve with time. Low sugar level in your blood – hypoglycaemia – occurs occasionally, one to two hours after meals. You feel weak, trembly and faint,

The possible operations (shown below) for peptic ulcers vary according to where the ulcer is situated. Most of them, however, involve the diversion of the food away from the affected area.

but these symptoms can be relieved rapidly by glucose tablets or any sugar, jam or guar gum.

Diarrhoea – which can feel very urgent – may occur after any stomach operation, but especially after a vagotomy. This affects one in ten people during the convalescent phase. Usually you get a repeating cycle of three or four days of watery diarrhoea, followed by a clear period. Taking codeine or loperamide will help. After you have returned to normal your motions may look pale. Iron-deficiency anaemia can follow, particularly after a partial gastrectomy operation. This is because of inadequate absorption of iron resulting from the operation or continuing slight blood loss from gastritis or oesophagitis which may occur as a complication. Biliary gastritis may develop from the reflux of bile through a drainage tube, with symptoms of discomfort, nausea, heartburn or vomiting. Dry meals and no cigarettes or alcohol may help, otherwise there is the final option of further surgery in extreme cases.

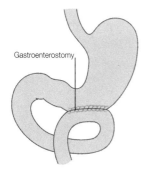
Gastroenterostomy

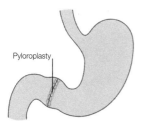
Pyloroplasty

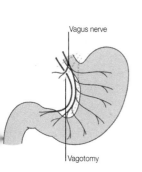
Vagus nerve

Vagotomy

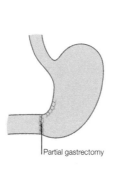
Partial gastrectomy

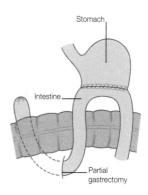
Stomach

Intestine

Partial gastrectomy

Q

77 I used to be
constipated
occasionally, but
since I have retired
this has become
more frequent. How
can I prevent this
becoming a real
nuisance?

You are constipated if you have to strain to pass a motion more often than one day in four, often miss two or three days in a row and produce dark brown, hard knobs of material.

If the constipation has come on recently, or become worse, you must go to see your doctor . In your case it seems that you have suffered from constipation on and off for years and now it is tending to become chronic.

Some causes of constipation include irritable bowel syndrome, under-active thyroid, diabetes, diverticular disease, after-effects of an operation – or pregnancy or dehydration, for instance because of feverishness. However, most commonly the cause lies in your lifestyle. Lack of exercise has this effect, and so does ignoring the call to go to the lavatory, eating irregular meals and having too little fibre. These are the items you must correct – for example increase your fibre intake – with foods such as wholemeal bread, bran cereal, baked beans and dried apricots. Remember also to drink plenty of water. If necessary use a laxative such as ispaghula husk, or if this is not effective, use a mild stimulant herbal laxative. Do not let your system grind to a halt, but reduce and stop the laxatives as soon as you can. Some medicines such as pain killers, antidepressants and contraceptive pills can cause constipation.

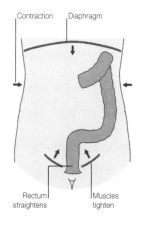

Contraction Diaphragm

Rectum straightens | Muscles tighten

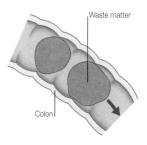

Waste matter

Colon

When passing a motion your diaphragm pushes down, your waist contracts and your abdominal muscles tighten which causes your rectum to straighten squeezing lumps of waste along the colon.

If you are constipated bludgeoning your bowel with harsh purgatives lessens its ability to respond in the long-term. It is wiser, therefore, to try the gentler, more natural herbal remedies, of which there is a wide selection. As a first choice try either ispaghula husk, senna pods, combined tea or orpsyllium seeds. Try letting five senna pods stand in water overnight, then drink the water. Ispaghula husk acts by swelling up, making your bowel feel full. It is often given with barberry or wahoo for the liver along with a general digestive stimulant like liquorice or dandelion. A tea is also made from equal parts of senna leaves, fennel seeds and chamomile flowers, infused for 15 minutes. One to three teaspoons of psyllium seeds are taken with sips of water, morning or evening. Some alternative tablets include either dandelion calamus, sweetflag root, seaweed and sarsaparilla or the 'Natural Herb Tablet' which includes holy thistle, aloes, fennel powder, myrrh powder, extract of skullcap, powdered lime flowers and valerian. Decoctions, herbs steeped in water overnight, can be made from black root, blue flag, buckthorn, cascara sagrada, dandelion root, turkey rhubarb or yellow dock. Combination powders contain turkey rhubarb and a trace of cayenne. Other preparations that are beneficial include barberry, liquorice, senna pods, slippery elm, buckthorn, fennel and elder. There are also some commercial preparations which you can buy over the counter. These are specially created to combat constipation in a safe and easy way.

Many herbalists also recommend a diet with no milk products and a teaspoonful of powdered agar-agar with meals, twice a day. Alternatively try yoghurt, crude black molasses and prunes soaked overnight or dandelion coffee and eat all the fibre-rich foods. Take supplements of vitamins A, B and C, and minerals potassium, calcium and zinc.

79 I often suffer from diarrhoea when I go on holiday. What precautions should I take to avoid this?

The causes of acute diarrhoea, including Traveller's Diarrhoea, include contamination of food by organisms or the toxins they produce, such as some strains of staphylococcus, campylobacter, clostridium and salmonella. It may also be produced by unusual strains of common germs such as E.coli. You may pick up 'gastroenteritis' viruses from other people without eating their food. Some medicines, for instance antibiotics, may also cause diarrhoea. Allergies, such as those to shellfish, is another cause.

Holiday-makers and travellers are susceptible to diarrhoea because they meet new and unaccustomed strains of organisms, but no special germ is responsible. When none is found a 'virus' is often blamed. Unfortunately it is almost impossible to avoid the problem. Prophylactic medication, to start before you go, is more likely to cause symptoms than prevent them. Drink plenty of fluids, with salt in a hot climate. Be meticulous about your hygiene, washing your hands after the toilet and before meals. Be aware of the hygiene of people handling food. Avoid raw fruit, salads, ice, ice-cream except an established make, and pre-prepared meat dishes. Meat and fish are safest either tinned or cooked thoroughly just before you eat them, for instance grilled steak or fried fish. If the water is suspect use bottled water for drinking and cleaning your teeth, or add chlorinating tablets. Water from the hot tap, if it is reasonably hot, is safer than from the cold, as it is likely to kill many organisms. An aperitif, and/or wine with your meal helps your stomach to resist infection by stimulating the production of acid, which is mildly anti-infective.

Q

80 What are the symptoms of a blockage of the intestine, and what can cause it?

Advance warning of a blocked intestine is given by increasing constipation – but as there are many other causes for this it is not the most reliable indicator. More reliable is colicky discomfort, which is apparent with a developing blockage in either the small or large intestine.

When a blockage has developed there is severe colic with restless shifting about in an attempt to ease the pain. Vomiting is an early symptom if the upper part of the intestine is affected, but occurs later if it is the colon that is affected. Conversely, constipation is an early symptom in a blocked colon, but later for the small intestine. Other symptoms include loud bowel sounds accompanied by cramp-like pain and a swelling of the abdomen. This swelling is different from the bloating of irritable colon or diverticular disease in that it does not decrease if you lie down. Faecal vomiting – that is bringing up material like diarrhoea – occurs in blockages very low in the colon, while passing neither motions nor wind, and no bowel sounds means complete obstruction – this is an emergency.

Common causes of blocked bowel are inflammation and oedema (swelling due to fluid in the tissues) – this may sometimes be relieved with steroid medication. Other causes include scarring from a disease such as Crohn's, tumours, either benign polyps or cancers, hernia, which may get twisted or strangulated and impacted motions. Occasionally the cause may be ileus, paralysis of the gut muscles in reaction to perforation or haemorrhage. Gallstone ileus is blockage of the small intestine by a big stone. Tumours outside the digestive system may also cause a block. Babies may have developmental abnormalities including an anus without an opening, and are subject to twisting and folding inwards of their intestines, volvulus and intussusception, respectively, which also cause blockage.

31

What is irritable bowel syndrome (IBS)? Who gets it, and what are the symptoms?

Irritable bowel syndrome is important, not because it is particularly dangerous, but because it affects so many of us – up to half those with gastroenterology disorders. It used to be called spastic colon or mucous colitis, but this was misleading. It does not affect only the colon, but any part of the digestive tract, from oesophagus to anus. It is a 'functional disease', which means that while there is no physical defect the digestion simply fails to function properly. This is why it proves so difficult to diagnose.

Women are more likely to suffer from IBS, as is anyone with a history of stomach-aches as a child. Other risk groups include people who have had a previous infection of the bowel, those who frequently use laxatives, and those who are anxious and have a general tendency to worry about things. Other factors include eating too much junk food, a low-fibre diet, and a gut that is over-sensitive to various common medicines. Further factors include a deficiency in lactase – an enzyme used for digesting milk, and any muscle disorder involving the involuntary muscles that control peristalsis. Alternatively you may have a life-long tendency for your bowel muscles to go into spasm when they should relax.

The symptoms are abdominal pain and constipation: these affect most sufferers. There may also be diarrhoea, with or without pain, bloating, odd appearance of motions ('rabbit pellets' – small and hard, thin ribbons or pencil-shaped, with a mix of different sizes and shapes), frequent motions, not necessarily runny, but urgent and mucus in the motions. Blood from a fissure or piles may streak the motions. There may be symptoms outside the digestive system including headache, dizziness, fatigue and poor concentration.

The pain of irritable bowel syndrome is widespread primarily because the affected organ, the colon, fills most of the abdominal area.

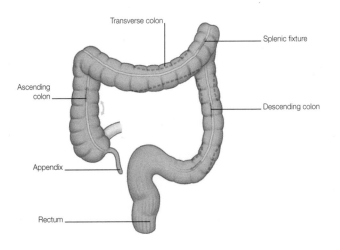

Transverse colon

Splenic fixture

Ascending colon

Descending colon

Appendix

Rectum

ABDOMINAL PAIN

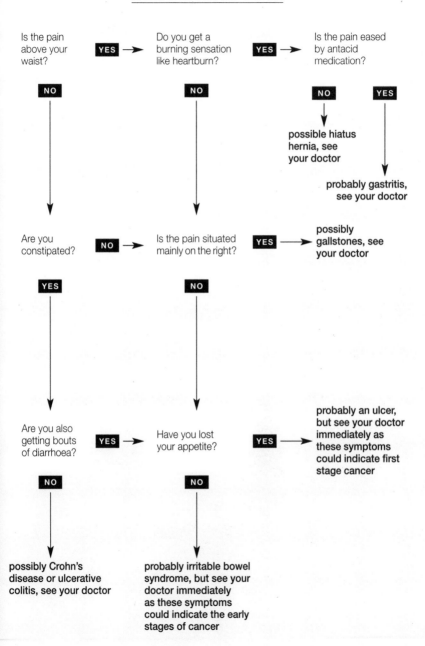

Is the pain above your waist? **YES** → Do you get a burning sensation like heartburn? **YES** → Is the pain eased by antacid medication?

NO → Is the pain eased by antacid medication? **NO** → possible hiatus hernia, see your doctor

YES → probably gastritis, see your doctor

Is the pain above your waist? **NO** → Are you constipated? **NO** → Is the pain situated mainly on the right? **YES** → possibly gallstones, see your doctor

NO (Is the pain situated mainly on the right?) ↓

Are you constipated? **YES** → Are you also getting bouts of diarrhoea? **YES** → Have you lost your appetite? **YES** → probably an ulcer, but see your doctor immediately as these symptoms could indicate first stage cancer

Are you also getting bouts of diarrhoea? **NO** → possibly Crohn's disease or ulcerative colitis, see your doctor

Have you lost your appetite? **NO** → probably irritable bowel syndrome, but see your doctor immediately as these symptoms could indicate the early stages of cancer

Q

82 What can be done to relieve irritable bowel syndrome (IBS)?

The first essential action is to have a thorough physical check by your doctor, so that you are sure that no serious disease has been overlooked. Next you require explanation and with it, reassurance. For example, you need to know that mucus in or with the motions is a sign of what you know already – that the bowel is irritated. You also need to know that cancer has no relation whatsoever to IBS, and that the pain you experience is not due to disease but to spasm in the muscles of a sensitive bowel.

You should start on a high-fibre diet, since it will be at least three months before you notice the benefit. Bran is comforting to the bowel, which cannot rest when it feels empty. Review your lifestyle, and try to reduce stress and deal with any potential causes of anxiety. Counselling or psychotherapy will help in many cases.

If you do need medication, anti-spasmodics are sometimes helpful. There are two principal types: musculotropics, which act either directly on the gut muscle, and include peppermint oil and mebeverine, and those which act via the nervous system, for example, dicyclomine. The latter, however, has side-effects including dry mouth, headache, dizziness and rash. The other type are called anxiolytics (relaxing medicines). These may be useful briefly if you are under strain, for example, buspirone or alprazolam, but they tend to be habit-forming.

Herbal remedies are often the most successful in the treatment of IBS. Only a few of those available are listed here. They include agrimony (an astringent), hops (colon analgesic) and ephedra (anti-sensitive) in equal parts; meadowsweet (an astringent) and chamomile (anti-inflammatory) in equal halves; also you could try calamus, goldenseal, or cranesbill in tablet form. Alternatively take five drops of oil of peppermint in a teaspoon of honey. For dietary supplements, try dandelion coffee and slippery elm gruel.

I've been told that inflammatory bowel disease (IBD) involves 2 illnesses, ulcerative colitis and Crohn's disease. What is the difference?

Ulcerative colitis is three times as prevalent as Crohn's disease, with 60 sufferers in every 100,000 compared with 30. In neither illness is the cause certain, but mycobacterium paratuberculosis is associated with Crohn's disease but not ulcerative colitis. Ulcerative colitis occurs at any age from infancy onwards but often starts in adolescence. Crohn's disease usually occurs between the ages of 10 and 40, but the peak ages are 20–29 and 70–79. In terms of personality ulcerative colitis sufferers tend to be extroverts, happy-go-lucky when they are well, but emotional under strain. People with Crohn's disease are often introverts, conscientious and reliable. The main symptom of ulcerative colitis is

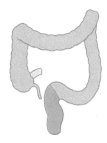

Ulceration of the rectum

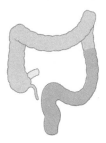

Ulceration of the rectum and descending colon

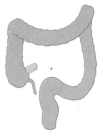

Ulceration throughout the colon

diarrhoea with blood and mucus, and in some, but not all, mild pain low down in the midline of the abdomen, and tenesmus (straining to pass a motion with nothing there). There is no general feeling of illness and no real weight loss.

Crohn's disease causes constant low abdominal pain, usually on the right and often cramps in the colon and rectum and loud tummy gurgles because of slight obstruction. There is also diarrhoea, but without blood and mucus. Loss of appetite occurs, you feel full after a few mouthfuls, and your food has no taste or smell, or tastes peculiar. Because of this and impaired absorption of nourishment in the small intestine, loss of weight is a major feature. You feel ill and your temperature is slightly raised. Children with Crohn's disease have their growth held back.

The sites of the diseases differ. In ulcerative colitis only the rectum and colon are affected. Crohn's disease can affect any part of the digestive tract, including the mouth and the anus. Ulcerative colitis only involves the mucous lining of the gut. Crohn's disease involves its whole thickness.

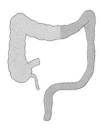

Ulceration from the splenic flexure

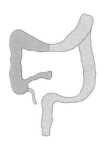

Ulceration of the ascending colon

Ulcerative colitis can occur anywhere throughout the digestive tract. However, the ulceration is normally found in specific sections rather than spread throughout.

Although ulcerative colitis and Crohn's disease have symptoms in common – diarrhoea and abdominal pain – the treatment differs.

For ulcerative colitis, during a severe attack you need bed-rest, plenty of fluids and a caring atmosphere – the victims of ulcerative colitis are often upset. Take no dairy products if you are allergic and follow a bland diet with smooth-textured, nourishing, cooked dishes with plenty of protein and a high calorie count. If a blood check shows anaemia you need an iron supplement and vitamin C to help its absorption, plus such non-irritating, natural sources such as corned beef, eggs, chocolate and treacle.

Medication for diarrhoea can be bought over the counter and includes codeine, which also relieve pain. Anti-spasmodics may help but is dangerous if the whole of the colon is affected. Sulphasalazine is mildly helpful in an attack, but really useful in preventing a relapse. Steroids, such as, prednisolone make you feel good but should not be used for more than six weeks with this disease, and do not prevent relapse. Surgery is necessary if the symptoms continue, or complications like perforation or haemorrhage arise. The usual operation is a colectomy, removal of the whole colon, with an ileostomy – an artificial anus.

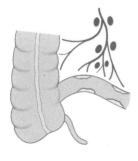

Crohn's disease not only affects the inner membrane of the digestive tract but also features enlarged lymph nodes surrounding the intestines.

For Crohn's disease the treatment for diarrhoea is the same as in ulcerative colitis, but differs otherwise. If you are anaemic, you may need vitamin B_{12} as well as iron by injection. You are generally ill-nourished because the small intestine is affected, the area where food is absorbed. Steroids are the linchpin of treatment and continue indefinitely. Antibiotics, for example metronidazole, are sometimes helpful. Immunosuppressants such as cyclosporin, methotrexate, and interferon sometimes help (salazopyrin is seldom helpful). Surgery involves either the removal of affected segments, or the whole colon.

Q

85 What is diverticular disease, and why is it becoming more common?

Diverticula are little pockets of gut lining which bulge out through the wall of the digestive tube. They can crop up anywhere along its length, but 90 per cent occur in the large bowel.

Diverticular disease comprises two conditions. Diverticulosis always comes first. It merely means the presence of diverticula – a minimum of three is needed to make the diagnosis, but usually there are many more. Diverticulitis involves inflammation and usually infection in some of the diverticula. While diverticulosis may cause some pain or discomfort it is often 'silent' and you do not know you have it. Diverticulitis, by contrast, is always painful and you may be feverish.

There are several reasons why it is becoming more frequent. It is a wear-and-tear disease, and as we are living longer there is more wear and tear. Women over 50 are the most vulnerable, and there are more women in the senior age groups. Changing lifestyle means technology is 'saving' us from the slightest effort – we can shop through the internet and, of course, drive instead of walk. Lack of exercise allows our muscles to become weak, making constipation more likely. Constipation is the key to diverticular disease. Straining to pass a hard motion increases the pressure inside the colon, forcing any weak parts to pop out as diverticula.

The modern Western diet is the main reason why diverticular disease affects 60 per cent of those over 60 in the most technologically advanced countries, but is almost unknown in the developing world. Soft, processed food, refined sugar, refined flour, and fats provide little residue. The colon requires a bulky filling which can be obtained by eating coarse, raw foods – fruit and vegetables and unrefined grain products.

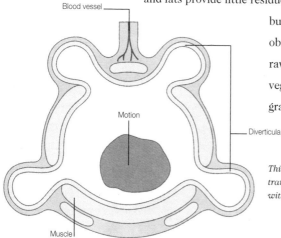

Blood vessel

Motion

Muscle

Diverticula

This illustration shows a transverse section of a colon with diverticular.

Q

86 How do I avoid
diverticular disease,
and what is the
treatment if I
do get it?

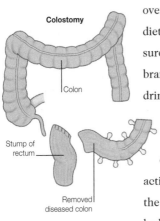

Colostomy

Colon

Stump of
rectum

Removed
diseased colon

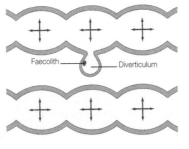

Faecolith — Diverticulum

Hartmann's operations. TOP:
*involves the removal of the
affected section of the colon.*
ABOVE: *A colon showing
internal pressure causing a
faecolith on the diverticulum.*

Most people with diverticular disease are unaware of it and only find out by chance. This is fortunate, since avoiding it is difficult. If you do have the disease the best you can do is to review your lifestyle and make adjustments. Are you overweight? Try to loose weight but eat a healthy diet, with the emphasis on your fibre intake. Make sure you include fruit, vegetables, wholemeal and bran. Do you drink much alcohol? Cut it back to one drink a day, two on your birthday. Do you get tense and anxious under stress? Fit in more leisure breaks and consider counselling. How much exercise do you take? Forty minutes of brisk activity (swim, gym or walk) three times a week is the minimum. The treatment for an acute attack is bed-rest, fluids, warmth and mental rest. Give your bowel a rest with a liquid diet and put high-fibre on hold for six to eight weeks. You may be given antibiotics and often pain-killers are prescribed. Also, anti-spasmodics may help, though these may have troublesome side-effects. In severe cases surgery may be needed if the disease develops complications. Continuing blood loss or perforation may require cutting out the affected part of the colon, or an abscess may need draining.

A friend told me he
might have to have
either an ileostomy
or a colostomy. What
are these? What
are they for?

An ileostomy and a colostomy are re-arrangements in the plumbing of the bowel. In both cases the motions come out through a new opening at the front of the abdomen instead of the anus. An ileostomy connects with the ileum, the last section of the small intestine, while a colostomy connects with the colon. The new opening is usually placed low down on the right for an ileostomy, and below and to the left of the navel for a colostomy. Very often a colostomy or ileostomy is a temporary measure and the continuity of the bowel, ending at the anus, is restored.

Sometimes these operations are needed urgently. An ulcer may penetrate right through the gut wall, spilling material into the abdomen, there may be intestinal obstruction, or toxic megacolon when the colon has become huge and paralysed. In cancer of the colon the affected section has to be removed. When the operation site has healed the remaining stump of colon can be joined up to the cut end, and the colostomy closed.

Less urgent reasons include chronic partial obstruction and complications like an abscess or a fistula (false passage into another organ) associated with Crohn's or diverticular disease. Essential equipment with an ostomy is a bag to collect the waste. Swimming, dancing and sex are all possible.

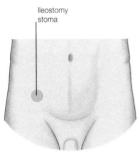

Ileostomy
stoma

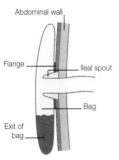

Abdominal wall

Flange

Ileal spout

Bag

Exit of
bag

An ileostomy removes the affected part of the intestine and replaces the need for a rectum and anus by the use of a bag situated on the right-hand side of the lower abdomen.

Recently I've been
suffering from severe
pain in the anus.
What are the most
likely causes of this?

Proctalgia fugax, literally 'fleeting pain in the back passage', causes the most severe pain in this area. It is so bad that the victim may faint, and it often wakes him or her from sleep. Recurrent attacks come without warning, each lasting 10–15 minutes. You feel you want to pass a motion, but there is nothing there, but later you may pass some wind, with increased pain. It is speculated that spasm in the rectum may be the cause, as it sometimes occurs with irritable colon syndrome. Another possibility is spasm and then release of the arteries in the region, producing an effect like migraine.

Strangulated pile or haemorrhoid is another cause of severe anal pain. If a pile prolapses – slips out of the anus – when you pass a motion and you are not able to push it in again, it can get stuck and constricted. It usually resolves with raising the foot of the bed, ice-packs and stool-softeners. Perianal Crohn's disease can affect young sufferers and comprises a Crohn's type inflammation with fissures and ulceration in the anus and surrounding skin. Passing a motion can be excruciating.

Other causes include a false passage into another organ caused by infection ulcerating through from an inflamed diverticulum, Crohn's disease opening into the anal area, or an anal fissure which is a deep crack in the skin of the anus.

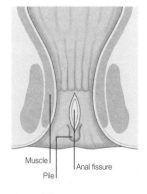

Muscle | Anal fissure
Pile |

An anal fissure can cause
severe pain and may indicate
further problems.

ANAL PAIN

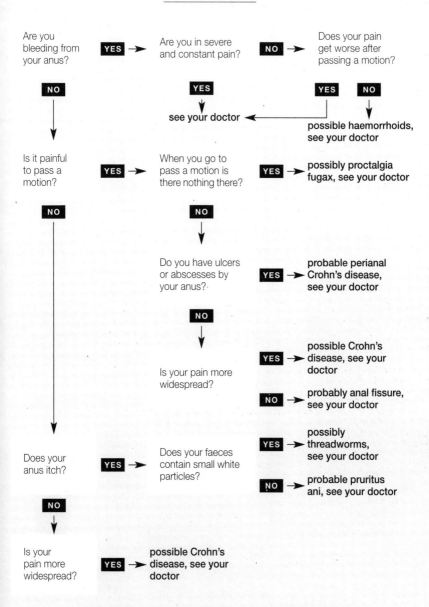

Are you bleeding from your anus? — **YES** → **Are you in severe and constant pain?** — **NO** → **Does your pain get worse after passing a motion?**

NO ↓

Are you in severe and constant pain? — **YES** ↓ **see your doctor**

Does your pain get worse after passing a motion? — **YES** → see your doctor / **NO** → **possible haemorrhoids, see your doctor**

Is it painful to pass a motion? — **YES** → **When you go to pass a motion is there nothing there?** — **YES** → **possibly proctalgia fugax, see your doctor**

NO ↓

When you go to pass a motion is there nothing there? — **NO** ↓

Do you have ulcers or abscesses by your anus? — **YES** → **probable perianal Crohn's disease, see your doctor**

NO ↓

Is your pain more widespread? — **YES** → **possible Crohn's disease, see your doctor** / **NO** → **probably anal fissure, see your doctor**

Does your anus itch? — **YES** → **Does your faeces contain small white particles?** — **YES** → **possibly threadworms, see your doctor** / **NO** → **probable pruritus ani, see your doctor**

NO ↓

Is your pain more widespread? — **YES** → **possible Crohn's disease, see your doctor**

You should always see your doctor with unexplained anal pain

Q
89 How do piles
develop? What
exactly are they,
and how can I avoid
getting them?

A pile is a fold of loose mucous membrane lying over the haemorrhoidal plexus, a cushion of tissue and veins just inside the anus. It is not, as we used to believe, a varicose vein of the back passage. The soft, thick membrane lining the anal canal has to have some slack to allow for a big motion to pass through a hole which is normally firmly closed by a ring of muscle – the anal sphincter. The chief reason for piles forming is the stretching and loosening of the redundant membrane by straining to pass a hard motion. Even the mild effort of passing a normal motion will, over the years, make the membrane more lax. Almost all the very elderly have piles, but they cause little trouble because the anal sphincter is loose, so there is no constriction. In younger people the powerful muscles of the region may squash or trap the pile and it is this damage to the delicate surface that causes bleeding.

To avoid getting piles, don't sit on the lavatory reading the paper and eat a high-fibre diet to avoid constipation. Don't let constipation develop: zap it promptly with bulk laxatives like ispaghula initially, and if these do not work try, temporarily, stimulating ones like senna and some herbal remedies. Ease a hard motion out with a glycerine suppository. Keep up an exercise programme, including abdominal exercises. Don't ignore the call to pass a motion.

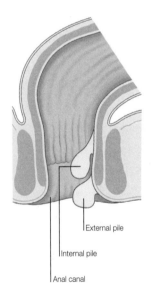

External pile

Internal pile

Anal canal

Haemorrhoids, or piles, may occur both internally and externally, when the internal pile falls out of the anus due to the loosening of the sphincter.

The treatment for piles varies according to the symptoms. These may be bleeding only, or you may feel the pile come down, out of the back passage, when you are passing a motion but it slips back by itself. In the next stage you have to push the pile back into your anus with your finger. Finally, it stays out all the time – or at least slides out even when you are not passing a motion, but walking or exercising. It may be difficult to get it back inside.

Treatments you can do at home are only suitable if your bleeding amounts to no more than a stain on the toilet paper, and the pile goes in again spontaneously. To avoid further problems shift to a high-fibre diet to avoid constipation, and a hot drink first thing helps wake up the bowels. Suppositories, creams and ointments are best avoided.

Outpatients treatments include injections of phenol and infra-red coagulation. Rubber band treatment to cut off the blood supply so the pile shrivels up, and cryosurgery – freezing – can both be used on large haemorrhoids, but they can be painful or lead to a nasty discharge for up to two weeks.

Day-patient treatment involves a general anaesthetic, reducing the pain of cryosurgery, while in-patient involves a haemorrhoidectomy – a 100 per cent guaranteed cure. You are in hospital two to three days, but off work for two to three weeks.

Q

91 I understand that uncontrollable leakage of the motions is more common than people let on. What are the possible causes?

Leaking from the back passage is under-reported because it is so embarrassing. Women who have had several children are the likeliest victims, but many older people find the sphincter muscle, which should close off the rectum, is now too weak.

If the muscles you control are weak you cannot wait, and may also leak when you laugh, cough, bend or walk. This is called stress incontinence. Another cause is injury: from difficult births, pelvic operations or anal dilatation. Impaction – blocking of the rectum by hard lumps of motion – which is particularly common in old people may also cause leakage. Loose, runny motions from any cause – even too many laxatives – can be difficult to contain. Dementia or a stroke can lead to incontinence as the nervous system deteriorates and the nerves fail to convey the message to go to the lavatory. Multiple sclerosis may cause incontinence by interfering with nervous control of the sphincter.

Any of the inflammatory bowel disorders can also cause stress incontinence, and so can large piles which are permanently down, or rectal prolapse where a part of the rectum is pushed out when you pass a motion. Finally, injuries to the spine affecting sensation and nervous control may cause you to loose your ability to control the sphincter as may spina bifida and other congenital abnormalities.

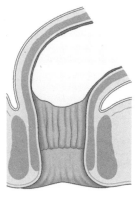

Motions can become impacted in the rectum causing constipation and severe pain.

92 What's the best way
of coping with
uncontrollable
leakage?

The good news about this disorder is that for sufferers who are otherwise fit, it can be cured. Your doctor will ask detailed questions, and whether you have a similar problem with holding your water.

To confirm the diagnosis the doctor must make a rectal examination (*see Q 42*). This will include proctoscopy – the use of an instrument to see a short way into the rectum. A pressure test (manometry) will be done to find out if the pressure at the anus is higher than in the rectum, which it must be to keep the motions in, and an electromyography will find any weak places in the sphincter. In severe cases a barium enema will reveal polyps, hidden prolapse or any similar disorder.

Treatments depend on the cause. Impaction can be relieved, and must be followed by regular emptying of the bowel using a glycerine suppository when necessary. Firming up motions that are too liquid, using medication may help and sometimes a high-fibre diet helps by increasing the bulk of the motions. In cases of muscular weakness, pelvic floor muscles can help so a general exercise programme is worthwhile. Surgical repairs to the sphincter and other muscles may be used in extreme cases. There are new treatments available using thigh muscle to fashion a new sphincter, and a plastic balloon device to encircle the anus.

Tumours & Cancer

We all worry about the possibility of getting cancer, and while there is no foolproof way to stop you getting the disease you can reduce the risk through a healthy diet, and the prognosis is better the earlier you catch the disease. This section explains the types of digestive cancers, how they are treated and what you can do to reduce the risk.

93 I have noticed a swelling under my jawbone, which seems to get bigger when I have something to eat. Is this a tumour?

The most likely cause of the swelling under your jaw is a salivary calculus in one of the submandibular glands in the region of your jawbone. There are three pairs of salivary glands (they produce saliva): the parotids, which are the mumps glands lying over your jaw joint; the sublingual, which lie under your tongue; and the submandibular, which are found under your jawbone.

The most common reason for a salivary gland to swell up is when a calculus (Latin for stone) forms in the gland and becomes lodged in the duct which carries the saliva from the gland into the mouth. Such stones are usually made of thickened saliva and calcium and are too hard to be secreted in the normal way in which saliva is deposited into your mouth. These therefore get stuck as they are pushed along with the saliva hence the blockage.

When a duct is blocked the relevant gland swells up with the trapped saliva, and, significantly, this happens particularly when your mouth would normally 'water'. This usually happens when you think of tasty food, see it, smell it, taste it or have it in your mouth. You can test whether your swelling is due to a salivary calculus by biting a segment of lemon. This would make a blocked gland get larger and hurt slightly because the gland produces saliver which it cannot excrete.

The cure is quick and easy – the doctor makes a small nick in the mucous membrane of the duct which is covering the stone and releases it. The cut heals quickly. The swollen salivary gland in such cases is sometimes known as a salivary tumour but this does not mean that it is cancerous.

'Mixed' salivary tumour is far less common. This is what is generally understood by the term 'tumour', that is to say tissues which are growing out of control. It can affect any of the salivary glands and can be diagnosed by a slow, painless enlargement of the gland, unaffected by eating, and comprised of connective tissue and tissue derived from skin, hence 'mixed'. This is a cancer that can vary from only slightly invasive to being more serious where it may involve the lymph glands in your neck. It calls for surgical removal, followed up in appropriate cases with radiotherapy. If your symptoms are not worsened by the lemon test you should go and see your doctor at once.

Q

94 My uncle has a stomach cancer. Is there any way to reduce the risk of getting it, and what are the symptoms?

The general anti-cancer ploys apply, including to stop smoking. You should eat plenty of fruit and vegetables, cut down on red meat, alcohol and refined grains like white bread and white rice. Search out anti-oxidants and make sure you eat plenty of walnuts, watercress, parsley, wheat sprouts and garlic. Take vitamins A, C and E supplements and the mineral, selenium. The predisposing causes involve things which are beyond our control, including nationality, having relatives with the disease, suffering from pernicious anaemia and belonging to blood group A. The last two suffer from a lack of stomach acid so steer clear of antacids.

A second line of defence against stomach cancer is to catch it very early. Symptoms to watch out for are loss of appetite, slight nausea and discomfort after meals. Have a check if you are over 40 when these crop up. Don't wait for the problems which come later to make an appearance: that is real pain and vomiting. Your friends will say you look pale and you will feel weak, while your weight drops away without you trying to lose it. A curious condition called acanthus nigricans occurs occasionally. It consists of black, velvety lesions like warts in the creases of your neck, groins or armpits. You may find your abdomen is getting distended – not due to fat but to fluid – called ascites.

The only cure for stomach cancer is an operation involving the removal of part, or in some cases, the whole of the stomach. There is a 95 per cent cure rate in Japan for tumours caught almost before they begin from their screening programme. In Europe and America we depend on the ordinary clinical symptoms to raise our suspicions, followed up by endoscopy – looking inside with a fibre-optic instrument. Even so, it is only when the abdomen has been opened that the surgeon can judge the feasibility of removing the tumour – a potential cure. This applies in about one case in three. Lesser operations are nevertheless worthwhile, for instance when a tumour is blocking the passageway into the duodenum causing distressing vomiting, or there is difficulty in swallowing from problems at the entrance. Both can be relieved. Ascites – the accumulation of fluid in the abdomen – can be drained off, and if an anti-cancer chemical such as methotrexate is instilled re-accumulation is delayed.

There are three forms of stomach cancer – a thin, all-over layer, the 'leather bottle' sort, which requires removal of the whole stomach, and less severe types; the cauliflower, which responds particularly well to treatment in older men, and the malignant ulcer, which is intermediate. If the cancer is considered inoperable, there are two other powerful treatments available – radiotherapy, which is particularly good at alleviating the pain and chemotherapy, which means taking a combination of two or three drugs.

When scientific medicine has little to offer, alternative therapies can help to improve a patient's quality of life – an aspect that can often be more important than merely prolonging life. They can help people to feel more comfortable, hopeful and at ease with themselves. Herbal remedies that have worked miracles for some include various teas; rosebay willowherb, star of Bethlehem and a mix of condurango, bayberry, liquorice and goldenseal.

96 I read that more and more people are suffering from cancer of the colon or rectum. Who is most likely to get one of these forms of cancer, and how can I avoid it?

In general it is men and women of aged 60 and over – peaking between 70 and 80 – who live in a technologically dominated culture who are the most likely to succumb to colo-rectal cancer. Figures show that Connecticut, USA is top of the league for this disease, with Los Angeles a close second, while it is never seen in Senegal. This is largely due to the Western diet which consists of too much fat, protein and processed foods, and too little of the fibre-rich raw fruit and vegetables, which provide the bulk the colon needs to function effectively.

Previous damage to the colon from diseases of the intestinal tract, including Crohn's disease and long-standing ulcerative colitis increases the risk. Having had colon cancer successfully removed once puts you at greater risk, while operations on the gallbladder or the urine tubes also make you more vulnerable. Colon cancer can run in the family and a condition involving multiple polyps – familial polyposis – is a particular risk because the polyps often become malignant.

To minimize your chances of getting colo-rectal cancer the first step is to review your lifestyle, especially in relation to what you eat (*see Q 100*). The anti-cancer diet of high-fibre and plenty of anti-oxidants is a must, as is cutting down on red meat, fat and alcohol. Supplements of vitamin D and calcium are considered especially important by some researchers, as is fish oil. Precautions also include taking immediate action if you notice a change in your bowel habit – and you are over 40. Sudden episodes of unexplained diarrhoea need reporting to your doctor and checking out, possibly with a barium enema or sigmoidoscope.

Polyps are small growths which appear on the intestine walls. These are generally benign but can become cancerous in certain cases.

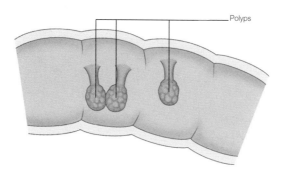
Polyps

Q

97

What is the
treatment
for cancer of the
colon and rectum?

It is vital that polyps of the large bowel are removed as they have the potential for becoming cancerous. This is can be done by surgery (colonoscopy) and a check with a colonoscope every few years. Where there are multiple polyps treatment is total removal of the whole colon, sometimes the rectum as well. Cancer of the colon can only be cured by surgery. For most, it involves the removal of the part of the colon that includes the tumour. The cut ends of the bowel are sewn together so that the motions can be passed via the anus as usual. If it is not feasible to cut out the cancerous area it is then by-passed. Even if there are secondaries in the liver, operating is well worthwhile because it relieves the symptoms. Cancer of the rectum means either removal of the upper part of the rectum so the continuity of the passage is preserved or a permanent colostomy with an artificial anus. Ultrasound and CT (computerized tomography) scans are used to monitor your progress, with colonoscopy every three years.

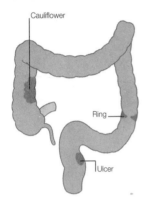

Cauliflower

Ring

Ulcer

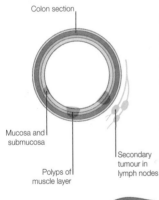

Colon section

Mucosa and
submucosa

Polyps of
muscle layer

Secondary
tumour in
lymph nodes

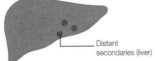

Distant
secondaries (liver)

*Cancer of the colon and rectum
can occur in many places along
the intestines and can lead to
secondary cancers outside the
intestine proper and in other
areas of the digestive tract.*

When an operation has effectively removed a cancer of the colon or rectum, you can look forward to restored health, and if a colostomy was not necessary, a normally functioning bowel. The number of unsuccessful operations is less than five per cent, and in some some centres less than two. Problems may include heart and chest disorders.

There is no part of the digestive tract, from mouth to anus, that is not subject to its own type of cancer. It is usually a carcinoma, a tumour derived from the lining membrane of the organ. In cases of the mouth, cancer commonly comes with an advance warning – a disorder called leukoplakia. It consists of firm white patches on the tongue, painless at first but later becoming malignant. This cancer is often related to smoking, alcohol and poor mouth hygiene. Tumour development of the oesophagus, too, is partly down to alcohol or tobacco, as well as very hot food. The most important symptom is difficulty swallowing, and the peak age for the illness is 60–70. If surgery is impracticable some relief is provided by implanting a plastic tube to carry fluids to the stomach. Cancer of the stomach is especially common in Japan and is most likely associated with diet, especially raw fish,

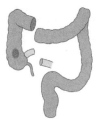

Cancer and removal of
the ascending colon

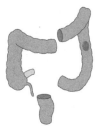

Cancer and removal of
the descending colon

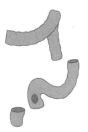

Cancer and removal
of the rectum

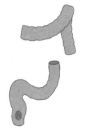

Cancer and removal of the
descending colon and rectum

different methods of preparing food, and nitrite food preservatives. Surgery gives excellent results – if it is performed early enough. The two main cancers of the duodenum and small intestine are lymphoma and carcinoma. The latter affects the duodenum and upper part of the intestine most frequently, often in people with coeliac or Crohn's disease, or polyposis. Bleeding often causes anaemia. In lymphoma the lymph glands are enlarged, and there is oedema – fluid swelling of the tissues. Colorectal carcinoma, cancer of the large bowel, is a very common cancer in the UK and USA, second only to lung cancer. It is often associated with chronic colitis, especially if the sufferer has the disease for ten years or more. Twenty-nine per cent of the tumours in colorectal cancer affect the sigmoid colon, 26 per cent the rectum – far more than any other parts of the large bowel. The common types of liver cancer are secondaries from tumours originally situated in the breasts, lungs or abdomen. Primary liver cancer, hepatoma, is uncommon in the West but frequently found in South Africa and South East Asia. Cancer of the gallbladder or of the bile ducts is rare.

*Cancer of the colon can affect
any part of the tract. This
means that any section may
have to be removed.*

What is the best
advice to give to
reduce the risk
of cancer in the
digestive system?

The risk for all types of cancer is influenced more by what you eat than any other factor. It is believed that a major effect of harmful substances we take in is likely to be in undermining our anti-cancer defences, rather than directly causing cancers to develop. The cancers most clearly related to diet are all in the digestive system. Apple alcohol (cider, calvados) is implicated, as is a shortage of niacin and zinc. Spirits and very hot food should be avoided. Protective factors for the stomach are fruits and vegetables, keeping food in the fridge, and plenty of vitamin C. Avoid adding salt to your food, salty foods, pickles – and smoking.

Animal fats and meat of all sorts appear to increase the cancer risk for the colon and beer for the rectum – take them in moderation. Wheat bran and fibre, are the best protective for this area – diluting and moving the harmful foods on through the colon faster. Brassica and other vegetables contain anti-cancer chemicals, also folate which inhibits genetic mutations. Beta-carotene is ineffective but soya, containing isoflavonoids, is beneficial. For the liver, the cancer risk is increased by various poisons, such as arsenic and thorotrast, also the male and female sex hormones and anabolic steroids, such as nandrolone. Industrial exposure in the metal and chemical trades has been linked with cancer of the pancreas, and food additives and preservatives are said to be a factor in one per cent of all cancers.

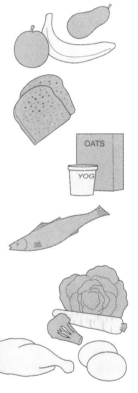

The anti-cancer diet should include lots of fresh fruit and vegetables, high-fibre alternatives, such as brown bread and cereals, and fresh fish and meat.

Useful Information

British Society of Gastroenterology
3 St Andrew's Place
Regents Park, London NW1 4LB
tel. 0207 387 3534
website:
http://www.bsg.org.uk

Digestive Disorders Foundation
3 St Andrew's Place
Regents Park, London NW1 4LB
tel. 0207 486 0341
website:
http://www.digestivedisorders.org.uk

Colon Cancer Concern
9 Rickett Street, London SW6 1RU
tel. 0207 387 9711
website:
http://www.coloncancer.org.uk

Colostomy Care Group
c/o The Irish Cancer Society
5 Northumberland Road, Dublin 4
tel: 01 668 1855
website:
http://www.irishcancer.ie

The Gastroenterological Society of Australia
website:
http://www.gesa.org.au

IBS Network
Northern General Hospital
Sheffield S5 7AU
answerphone: 0114 2611531
email: Penny@ibsnetwork.org.uk

Cancer BACUP
3 Bath Place
Rivington Street, London EC2A 3JR
Tel. 0207 696 9003
Fax 0207 6969 9002
www.cancerbacup.org.uk

South African Natural Health Network tel: 021 762 5612
website:
http://www.naturalhealth.co.za

Natural Health Society of Australia
28/541 High Street
Penrith, NSW 2750
tel: 02 4721 5068

FURTHER READING

GOMEZ, J., *Living with Crohn's Disease,* Sheldon, 2000
—*Positive Options in Crohn's Disease,* Hunter House, 2000
—*Coping with Gallstones,* Sheldon, 2000
—*Coping Successfully with Diverticulitis,* Wellhouse, forthcoming

JONES, D. J. (Ed.), *ABC of Colorectal Diseases* 2nd Edn, BMJ Books, 1999

ELIAS, E., HAWKINS, C., *Lecture Notes on Gastroenterology,* Blackwell, 1985

STEWART TRUSWELL, A., *ABC of Nutrition* 3rd Edn, BMJ Books, 1999

VANN JONES, J., TOMSON, C., *Essential Medicine,* Churchill Livingstone, 1998

GUYTON, A. C., *Textbook of Medical Physiology,* 7th Edn, Saunders, 1990

EDWARDS, C., BOUCHIER, I., *Davidson's Principles and Practice of Medicine,* Churchill Livingstone, 1992

HOFFMAN, DAVID, *Healthy Digestion – A Natural Approach,* Newleaf, 2001

BERKSON, LINDSEY, *Healthy Digestion in the Natural Way,* Wiley, 2000

BOLEN, BARBARA BRADLEY, *Breaking the Bonds of Irritable Bowel Syndrome*, New Harbinger Publications, 2000

TRICKETT, SHIRLEY, *Irritable Bowel Syndrome and Diverticulosis A Self-Help Plan,* Thorsons, 1999

THOMPSON, W. GRANT, *Angry Gut Coping with Colitis and Crohn's Disease*, Plenum Publishing, 1993

ROSENTHAL, M. SARA, *50 Ways to Prevent Colon Cancer,* Laura Purday, 2000

HALL, LINDSEY, COHN, LEIGH, *Bulimia: A Guide to Recovery,* Gurze Designs & Books, 1999

LEVENKRON, STEVEN, *Anatomy of Anorexia,* W. W. Norton, 2000

Index